THE MIND DIET

2ND EDITION

THE MIND DIET

2ND EDITION

A Scientific Approach to Enhancing Brain Function
and Helping Prevent Alzheimer's and Dementia

MAGGIE MOON, MS, RD

Foreword by Jon Artz, MD

Published by:
Ulysses Press
PO Box 3440
Berkeley, CA 94703
www.ulyssespress.com

ISBN: 978-1-64604-724-6
Library of Congress Control Number: 2024934549

Printed in the United States
10 9 8 7 6 5 4 3 2 1

Managing editor: Claire Chun
Project editor: Renee Rutledge
Proofreader: Sherian Brown
Index: S4Carlisle
Front cover design: Rebecca Lown
Cover artwork: © Sea Wave/shutterstock.com, egg © jerrysa/shutterstock.com
Layout: Winnie Liu

IMPORTANT NOTE TO READERS: This book has been written and published strictly for informational and educational purposes only. It is not intended to serve as medical advice or to be any form of medical treatment. You should always consult your physician before altering or changing any aspect of your medical treatment and/or undertaking a diet regimen, including the guidelines as described in this book. Do not stop or change any prescription medications without the guidance and advice of your physician. Any use of the information in this book is made on the reader's good judgment after consulting with his or her physician and is the reader's sole responsibility. This book is not intended to diagnose or treat any medical condition and is not a substitute for a physician.

This book is independently authored and published and no sponsorship or endorsement of this book by, and no affiliation with, any trademarked brands or other products mentioned within is claimed or suggested. All trademarks that appear in ingredient lists and elsewhere in this book belong to their respective owners and are used here for informational purposes only. The author and publisher encourage readers to patronize the brands mentioned and pictured in this book.

For Mom, Youjae Kang Moon,
and
Dad, Dr. In Eon Moon

CONTENTS

FOREWORD

This is my twenty-fifth year caring for patients as a board-certified adult neurologist and neurophysiologist. I have developed over the last two decades an unwavering commitment to better understanding the role of lifestyle factors in preventing diseases in my specialty. Nutrition is one of the foundations for promoting and maintaining a healthy existence, and science has clearly time and again validated the relevance and contributions of food to both positively and negatively impacting one's health. It was time for Maggie to update her widely known and read *The MIND Diet,* and it is my honor to address you—the reader—as a brain-health practitioner who is a strong believer in what it has to offer you.

As a cognitive health specialist who maintains a focus on advocacy for brain-health prevention strategies and lifestyle interventions, I believe the 2nd edition of *The MIND Diet* meets my strict criteria for an easy-to-understand, evidence-based, and reliable resource that can make a positive and enduring change in health. From an academic perspective, I recognize the potential impact this book can have on my patients' health, specifically for individuals who are noticing changes in their thinking and memory, which fall under the umbrella term of "cognition."

Consistent with the initial edition, the 2nd edition is a manifesto on the relevance of how influential nutrition is for one's health and healthy aging across the lifespan. I strongly believe from my experience and understanding of brain science that this updated version of *The MIND Diet* is relevant for any individual who wants not only to understand how to become brain healthy, but to have the ingredients (both literally and figuratively) to optimize brain function and reduce the risk of developing brain-related ailments, including Alzheimer's and Parkinson's disease.

Maggie received considerable feedback from her readers over the last eight years and has used many of these suggestions to enhance the value of this 2nd edition. This included creating a diverse selection of over sixty globally inspired recipes, an all-new FAQ section, updated and expanded tip sheets, and new biomedical research findings from the 150-plus studies published since the initial MIND studies, covering a wide range of topics including cognitive performance, healthy aging, cardiovascular health, type 2 diabetes, and more. Maggie was clearly invested in improving this guidebook with her readers' health as her highest priority.

You will quickly recognize the depth and breadth of Maggie's talent and skill in explaining the latest evidence on nutrition science. She has upgraded an already-great book with a blueprint for a healthy way of eating by emphasizing the power of whole foods and their nutrients in promoting health and wellness.

The power of nutrition and its role as a pillar for cognitive health is fully apparent in Maggie's 2nd edition. I believe *The MIND Diet* "2.0" is a critical resource for anyone and everyone that desires to take their brain health seriously.

In good health,
Jon Artz, MD
Board-certified neurologist and
cohost of the *Let's Talk Brain Health* podcast

PREFACE

Dear Reader,

If you're new to the MIND diet, it's helpful to know "MIND" is an acronym for a dietary pattern created to study how what we eat affects our brain health. It stands for Mediterranean-Dietary Approaches to Stop Hypertension Intervention for Neurodegenerative Delay, and research suggests following it is associated with better cognitive performance and a reduced risk of brain diseases.

More than 150 new research papers have been written about the MIND diet since the first research on it was published in 2015. In that time, I've grown older and my parents have entered their eighties, mostly in good health, I'm happy to report. But if we're fortunate to see the years go on, there's no denying that we must provide more care and maintenance to the brain and body. I've seen and felt this firsthand. Nutrition isn't the only piece of the successful aging puzzle, but it's a fundamental one. To that end, I'm sharing important updates from the new MIND diet research studies—which are strongest in the areas of memory, cognition, and dementia prevention, but I'll also cover what we now know about the MIND diet for cardiovascular health, healthy aging, Parkinson's disease, and mental health.

Since the first edition of this book, I completed culinary school and took the journey from fussy foodie to practical home cook. Fun fact: My husband and I cooked all of our meals for two years during the COVID-19 pandemic. He became an excellent sous-chef and more recently made most of our meals while I was working on updating this book. All that to say, while we save "fussy" for special occasions, we make most of our meals quick, simple, fresh, and delicious. It's with this sensibility that I've created all new recipes for this edition. But simple doesn't mean boring, and you can look forward to a dash of global flavors inspired by my childhood in a Korean American home and my world travels.

Like the original edition, this book is about eating right to keep your brain younger for longer. The recommendations continue to be based on the latest science on which foods and nutrients benefit and harm brain function, while staying grounded in two proven diets that have been studied for many decades and practiced, in good health, for centuries. Namely, the Mediterranean diet and Dietary Approaches to Stop Hypertension (DASH), which are the "M" in MIND.

The science is there for you, but if you want to skip straight to the updated tips, tools, recipes, and resources, do what's right for you. This book is for you, reader, to use in whatever way serves you best right now.

As a nutrition educator by training, I hope this book serves as an approachable guide to the science and foods for optimal brain health, served up in a culturally humble way. Ultimately, my hope is to support and empower you until you're eating well, living well, and thriving as effortlessly as we breathe.

Be well,
Maggie Moon, MS, RD

INTRODUCTION

The world is aging. In 2020, adults over 60 outnumbered children under 5,[1] and one in every six people in the United States was over 60[2] (it will be one in five by 2030). Worldwide, one in six people will be over 60 by 2030, and this represents one of the largest demographic shifts of our lifetime.

With age comes wisdom that should be respected, appreciated, and cherished. However, with age also comes an increased risk of cognitive decline and dementia. Today in the US, one in nine adults over 45 experiences subjective cognitive decline, which could be an early sign of dementia in later years; and one in nine over 65 lives with Alzheimer's dementia. But dementia is not a normal part of aging.

Research suggests that what we put on our plates can help or hinder how well we think, learn, and remember. Our cognitive health is essential for independent living and thriving in every season of life. The brain is the keeper of our memories, but also the conductor of how well we reason, make sound choices, and even navigate physical spaces. There's no reason to let cognitive decline or dementia rob us of good years, and a healthy diet is an essential part of the solution.

---

1 World Health Organization, "Ageing and Health," October 1, 2022, https://www.who.int/news-room/fact-sheets/detail/ageing-and-health.

2 US Census Bureau, "2020 Census: 1 in 6 People in the United States Were 65 and Older," May 25, 2023, https://www.census.gov/library/stories/2023/05/2020-census-united-states-older-population-grew.html.

The best time to start eating for brain health is now, especially since it is well-accepted that changes to the brain and body start 20-plus years before memory loss and other symptoms appear.[3] The MIND diet is one approach that may help, and it's unique because it is a research-backed eating pattern developed specifically for brain health. Following the MIND diet is associated with slowing down brain aging by up to 7.5 years and reducing the risk of Alzheimer's by up to 53 percent.[4] It has also shown benefits for healthy aging, premature death, heart health, type 2 diabetes, and mental health. It has components of the well-researched Mediterranean and Dietary Approaches to Stop Hypertension (DASH) diets, which are known for being heart-healthy. However, the specific mix of foods in the MIND diet appear to offer superior brain health support.

The MIND diet, which was developed in the US, includes 15 types of food, including five types of foods to limit, but twice as many to enjoy. The best foods for your brain include leafy green vegetables, nuts, beans, berries, poultry, fish, whole grains, and olive oil. The foods to limit (though total elimination is not mandatory) are red meat, butter and stick margarine, whole-fat cheese, pastries and sweets, and fried fast food. The MIND diet has since been adapted by researchers to two non-Western eating patterns with culturally appropriate updates, but they have more in common than not. These alternate takes on the MIND diet from Korea and China are briefly described in this book, noted as K-MIND and cMIND, respectively.

You can expect this second edition of *The MIND Diet* to provide an update on the past nine years of research findings, along with

---

3 Livingston et al., "Dementia Prevention, Intervention, and Care," *Lancet* 396, no. 10248 (2020): 413–446, doi: 10.1016/S0140-6736(20)30367-6.

4 Morris et al., "MIND Diet Associated with Reduced Incidence of Alzheimer's Disease," *Alzheimer's & Dementia Journal*, 11, no. 9 (2015): 1007–1014, doi: 10.1016/j.jalz.2014.11.009; Morris et al., "MIND Diet Slows Cognitive Decline with Aging," *Alzheimer's & Dementia Journal* 11, no. 9 (2015): 1015–1022. doi: 10.1016/j.jalz.2015.04.011.

updated tip sheets, worksheets, a new frequently asked questions section, and all-new recipes.

To set the stage, part one of this book explains the basics of the brain and mental fitness, as well as the science behind the MIND diet, in an approachable and understandable way. It summarizes the research backing the recommendations to seek or avoid certain foods and nutrients for brain health.

Next, part two of the book will guide you through how to create your own MIND diet plan, including what to eat, how much, and how often. You'll find helpful worksheets for meal planning, keeping track of your progress, and overall lifestyle recommendations for brain health.

Part three of the book features profiles on the brain-healthy foods that form the foundation of the MIND diet, from seasonality and culinary uses to fascinating historical background. I provide guidance and strategies for choosing the healthiest options when confronted with foods from the brain-harming food groups. I also provide tip sheets that deliver practical information at a glance to help you get started and take the guesswork out of navigating the MIND diet, as well as a fully updated frequently asked questions section that addresses the top questions I've received over the years.

Part four brings the MIND diet to life through 60-plus all-new recipes that offer delicious and nutritious options for smoothies, small plates, snacks, salads, soups, mains, sides, desserts, and even sips and elixirs.

This book is about hope, prevention, and taking positive action today to slow cognitive decline and minimize the risk of Alzheimer's disease down the road.

PART ONE

The Science of the MIND Diet

The science of the MIND diet is an active area of study that's more than 150 studies strong at the time of this writing. To better understand the science, it's helpful to understand basic brain anatomy and key concepts such as cognition, cognitive decline, dementia, Alzheimer's disease, and how mental fitness is tested.

Part one of this book reviews seminal studies demonstrating the diet's potential to cut Alzheimer's risk in half and slow cognitive decline. The focus then shifts to the broad health benefits of the MIND diet, including its positive impact on cognitive health, heart health, diabetes, metabolic syndrome, mental health, Parkinson's disease, healthy aging, and reducing premature death.

Research on how the MIND diet has been adapted to cultures outside the US, with specific insights into results from Korea, China and France, reveals how eating for brain health can include culturally relevant foods. The final section of part one explains the science behind specific foods and nutrients that impact brain health and provides a wide range of examples of brain-healthy foods.

CHAPTER 1
THE BRAIN

Super-Basic Brain Overview

What follows is a very basic orientation to the brain and general cognitive functions that will be relevant in this book. It is by no means comprehensive or even very detailed. Simple information about various sections of the brain will be explained in approachable language. For example, rather than discuss the anterior and posterior brain, words like "front" and "back" will be used.

After establishing a basic framework for how the brain works, this chapter will explore how the brain changes with cognitive decline, dementia, and Alzheimer's disease.

Brain Basics

The brain has three main parts. The largest part of the brain is called the cerebrum, and it handles higher functions like reasoning, learning, emotions, speech, fine motor control, correctly interpreting touch, vision, and hearing, and of course, memory. The other two parts are smaller and sit under the cerebrum. They're called the cerebellum and brainstem, and they regulate basic functions like breathing, digestion, body temperature, and balance. When this book discusses brain health, it is referring to the cerebrum.

The brain has two sides—left and right—called hemispheres. Each hemisphere has four sections, one in front, one in back, and two in the middle stacked on top of each other. These sections are called lobes, and there are eight total.

Each lobe is affiliated with a certain set of functions. Lobes are not independent, though. It's important to recognize that just like no individual is an island, no lobe can act alone. Brain-imaging studies have shown how multiple parts of the brain are active at the same time during any given task.

The front lobe, aptly called the frontal lobe (they aren't all named with as much common sense), is the most advanced area of the brain. It receives information gathered through the senses (sight, touch, taste, hearing, smell) and spatial awareness (e.g., balance and movement), and is in charge of planning, short-term memory (working memory), understanding abstract ideas, inhibiting behaviors that may be emotionally or socially inappropriate, voluntary movement, and expressive language. These complex planning behaviors are associated with activity in the front part of the frontal lobe, called the prefrontal cortex, which lies just behind the forehead.

The lower middle lobe, called the temporal lobe, plays a major role in hearing, understanding language, memory, and learning and retaining information. There are upper, middle, and lower regions that are technically called superior, medial, and inferior. The medial temporal lobe (MTL) includes the hippocampus, which is involved with forming long-term memories and spatial navigation abilities. When it's damaged, the result is memory loss and disorientation.

The upper middle lobe is called the parietal lobe and is the key player in making sense of what the body touches. It's also involved in spatial thinking, such as rotating objects in your mind, being able to store ideas of movement, and controlling your intention to move. This part of the brain comes in handy in dance classes. Also, like the frontal lobe, it's involved in short-term memory.

The last and fourth section is at the back of the brain. This back lobe is called the occipital lobe. This area of the brain is farthest from the eyes, and yet, is the primary center for making sense of what you see. It is extremely important in vision.

Just below the back lobe is an area called the cerebellum, which is important to know because it has more neurons than any other part of the brain. It has many connections to the frontal lobe and most other areas of the brain. It's involved in learning and coordinating movement.

The Hungry Brain

The brain is one of the body's hungriest organs, especially for its size. The brain makes up only 2 percent of body weight but consumes up to 20 percent of daily calories and oxygen. The brain's preferred energy source is glucose, which it gets when the food we eat is broken down and some of the glucose is transported in blood, across the blood-brain barrier, and into brain cells. It has a high metabolism and uses up nutrients quickly.

Not only is the brain hungry for energy (calories), it's also hungry for antioxidants. The brain has a high need for antioxidants because it's such a metabolically active organ, which creates an abundance of oxidative molecules called free radicals (unstable molecules that damage cells). As you can imagine, this makes the brain particularly susceptible to oxidative stress, a result of having more free radicals than antioxidants to neutralize them. Oxidative stress causes damage to the brain tissue. In fact, a theory in the field of brain disorders is that the brain needs to be saved from oxidation and inflammation via protective plant compounds with antioxidant and anti-inflammatory properties (e.g., vitamins E, C, and A, flavonoids and other polyphenols, manganese, copper, selenium, zinc, enzymes, and more).

There are two kinds of antioxidants the body uses: enzymes made by the body (endogenous antioxidants) and nutrients from food (dietary antioxidants). The antioxidant enzymes the body creates can prevent toxic substances from being created in the first place, and antioxidant nutrients from food can neutralize the damaging consequences of oxidation, such as free radicals. The brain doesn't have as many endogenous antioxidant enzymes at its disposal as other parts of the body, which means dietary antioxidants have a big role to play. This is one reason good nutrition and healthy eating is so important to maintaining a healthy brain.

The Fat Brain

Similar to the rest of the body, most of the brain is water (about 75 percent). However, take away the water and you're left with brain matter, 60 percent of which is fat (also known as lipids). Fats are an essential structural component of neurons. It's no surprise, then, that the brain needs healthy fats to function properly, from facilitating better blood flow to improving memory and mood. Neurons communicate through a signaling system that gets updated when a new supply of fatty acids is available.

The body produces all the saturated fat it needs, but some fats need to come from the diet. Namely, essential polyunsaturated omega-3 and omega-6 fats. The American diet typically supplies enough omega-6 fats, but not enough omega-3s, which come from fish, nuts, and seeds.

The most metabolically active fat in the brain is a polyunsaturated type of fat called omega-3 docosahexaenoic acid (DHA), which is found in fatty fish like salmon. The body can also convert omega-3 alpha-linolenic acid (ALA), which comes from plant foods like flaxseed, perilla seeds, and walnuts, into DHA. That means the body doesn't technically require outside sources of DHA, but it's helpful since it only converts about half a percent of ALA to DHA.

As different fats are digested and absorbed, cholesterol is transported around the body in various forms, such as LDL cholesterol (sometimes called "bad" cholesterol) and HDL cholesterol (sometimes called "good" cholesterol). Cholesterol is an essential part of healthy cell membranes, and plays a role in hormone and vitamin D production. The role of cholesterol in Alzheimer's disease isn't fully clear, but studies have found that higher levels of LDL cholesterol is linked to more Alzheimer's disease–associated plaque in the brain (amyloid plaques).

What Is Cognition?

To understand what cognitive decline is, it's important to first identify just what cognition is. Cognition includes how we think, learn, and remember. Cognition affects how a person understands the world and acts within it, and it includes all the mental skills needed to carry out simple and complex tasks alike, from locking the front door to analyzing a scientific report. To elaborate, cognition is a word that describes the process of receiving sensory inputs (e.g., what we see, read, touch, taste, feel, smell, or hear), and transforming those inputs into their most important components (reduction), filling in gaps (elaboration), remembering (storing and recovering memories), and using the inputs to interact with the world around us, understand language, solve problems, and more.

According to the National Institute on Aging, a division of the National Institutes of Health in the U.S. Department of Health & Human Services:

Cognition is the ability to think, learn, and remember. It is the basis for how we reason, judge, concentrate, plan, and organize. Good cognitive health, like physical health, is very important as we get older, so that we can stay independent and keep active. Some declines in cognition and memory with age are normal, but sometimes they can signal problems.

Types of cognitive functions include perception, attention, memory, motor skills, language, visuospatial processing, and executive functioning, as further explained below.

- **Perception** is how our senses recognize and process information. It's what happens when we receive sensory inputs.
- **Attention** is the ability to continue to concentrate on something while filtering out competing thoughts or sensory stimulation in the environment. It includes reduction skills.
- **Memory** can be short term or long term. Short-term memory can be as short as 20 seconds and might be used when reading a step in a recipe before doing it, for example, while long-term memory is just that and stores memories for years and years.
- **Motor skills**, not often thought of as a cognitive ability, definitely use brain power, and the loss of these skills can be part of the challenges of cognitive decline. These are the skills used to move our muscles, from walking and cooking to dancing or playing sports, including the ability to manipulate objects such as swinging a pickleball paddle or using a pen.
- **Language skills** are what allow the brain to understand (translate sounds into words) and use language (generate verbal responses).
- **Visuospatial skills** include the ability to see objects and understand the spatial relationship between them. For example, being able to tell how far apart two pencils are when placed near each other, and whether they are lying at the same or different angles. These skills are also used when mentally rotating a shape (helpful when organizing a full refrigerator or packing a suitcase).
- **Executive functioning** can also be thought of as reasoning skills and includes the ability to plan and do things. These abilities include using flexible thinking modes, empathetically imagining what someone else likes or dislikes, anticipating an outcome based on past experience, identifying a problem and

finding solutions, making choices, using short-term memory to receive information just long enough to use it (working memory), being self-aware of emotions enough to manage them, breaking down complex ideas or actions into small steps and putting them in the right order of what needs to get done first (this is what a home cook does when they think through how to make a recipe), and focusing in a manner that can eliminate inner and outer distractions.

What Is Cognitive Decline?

Cognitive decline is a decrease in cognitive abilities over time. Some age-related cognitive decline is considered "normal," including slower thinking and having a harder time with prolonged attention, multitasking, short-term memory, and word finding. On the other hand, vocabulary, verbal reasoning, and synthesizing information from diverse sources of information is often maintained or improved.

The normal aging brain may show signs of cognitive wear and tear due to a loss of gray matter volume and changes to white matter. Gray matter fills 40 percent of the brain, and white matter fills the remaining 60 percent. Gray matter is where all the processing goes on; white matter allows different gray areas to communicate with one another and with other parts of the body. If gray matter is like a factory, then white matter is the trucking fleet that transports goods from one factory to another, or from factory to store. It seems that when it comes to age-related cognitive decline, the issue is not black and white, it's gray and white.

As a part of normal aging, the amount of gray matter starts to go down after age 20, especially in the prefrontal cortex, but also in the hippocampus. Scientists believe this decrease might be due to dying neurons. A protein called beta-amyloid, which has been found in all people with Alzheimer's dementia, can kill neurons. Beta-amyloid is also found in 20 to 30 percent of normal adults, which may, but doesn't necessarily, predict that they'll develop Alzheimer's disease. Another explanation is that neurons grow smaller and the number of connections between them also decreases. These decreases are very well documented in older adults. With aging, neurons become simpler, shorter, and less connected to other neurons.

White matter shrinks more than gray matter as we get older. Similar areas of the brain have shown 16 to 20 percent losses of white matter but only 6 percent of gray matter loss. The consequences of these normal changes to the brain over time are small and shouldn't get in the way of daily activities.

In contrast to age-related cognitive decline, a condition called mild cognitive impairment (MCI) is more serious and is a risk factor for Alzheimer's disease. However, having mild cognitive impairment doesn't always lead to Alzheimer's disease and presents an opportunity to make important lifestyle changes. MCI is a condition that affects memory and thinking (e.g., planning, organizing, judgment) enough that it's noticeable, but not to the point that it interferes with daily life. Some causes of cognitive impairment, such as medication side effects, vitamin B12 deficiency, and depression, are treatable.

A newer designation of subjective cognitive decline (SCD) represents an even earlier opportunity for intervention. It is defined by the Centers for Disease Control as "self-reported confusion or memory problems that have been happening more often or getting worse in the past 12 months."

What Is Dementia?

Dementia literally means "without mind" (de = without; mentia = mind). Dementia is a set of symptoms but not a disease of its own. It's a term used to describe symptoms that can be caused by brain disorders such as Alzheimer's disease or a stroke. Symptoms of dementia include problems with memory, thinking, language, or social skills, and uncharacteristic behavior changes. Getting older doesn't cause dementia, though dementia is more common in older adults. The occasional forgetfulness, having trouble recalling a word, or any of these symptoms could be a normal part of aging without being related to dementia. The difference is when the symptoms start to get in the way of everyday life, or activities of daily living (ADL); for example, when symptoms become disruptive to working, getting dressed, or making meals. Cognitive impairment is also associated with difficulty managing instrumental activities of daily living (IADL). These activities are associated with multiple mental processes, which is why they are sensitive to cognitive decline. They can provide another signal to pay more attention to brain health.

Examples of ADL:

- **Bathing**—washing yourself, including getting in and out of the tub or shower.
- **Dressing**—putting on and taking off clothes, shoes, braces, artificial limbs.
- **Going to the toilet**—getting to and from, on and off, and using the toilet.
- **Getting around the house**—sometimes called transferring. This refers to getting in and out of bed, chairs, or a wheelchair.
- **Continence**—being able to control bowel and bladder functions.
- **Eating**—eating and drinking enough to meet nutritional needs.

Examples of IADL:

- Managing finances
- Managing medications
- Using a phone
- Preparing hot meals
- Shopping for groceries
- Using a map
- Driving a car

By mid-century, approximately a quarter of the US population will be 65 years and older, and more than one in three of this older population is projected to develop dementia. The rate of dementia rises drastically with advancing years. According to the 2024 Alzheimer's disease facts and figures report from the Alzheimer's Association, 27 percent of Alzheimer's cases are in adults ages 65 to 74, while 73 percent are in adults over 75. Alzheimer's currently affects 5 percent of 65- to 74-year-olds, 13 percent of 75- to 84-year-olds, and 33 percent of those 85 years old and up.[5] Further, people of color are projected to be disproportionately affected.

There are over 50 different conditions associated with dementia, but the most common cause of dementia is Alzheimer's disease, which accounts for 60 to 80 percent of all cases of dementia. Lewy body disease (abnormal protein clumps in brain cells), hardening arteries (arteriosclerosis) in the brain, and stroke are also common causes of dementia. Other diseases that can cause the symptoms of dementia are Parkinson's disease, Huntington's disease, HIV infection, head injury, severe depression, and Creutzfeldt-Jakob disease.

There are also nondisease causes of dementia symptoms. The National Institutes of Health indicates that dementia-like symptoms could be the result of medications, metabolic problems, nutritional deficiencies, infections, poisoning, brain tumors, lack of oxygen to the brain, and heart and lung problems.

Most dementias are irreversible. However, there are exceptions to this rule. Some forms of dementia can be stopped or even reversed if caught soon enough. These include dementia-like symptoms caused by vitamin deficiencies, brain tumors, chronic alcoholism, and some medications. For the remaining forms of dementia, current treatment options may help with symptoms but do offer a cure. This is why health professionals are focused on prevention.

---

5 Alzheimer's Association, "2024 Alzheimer's Disease Facts and Figures," https://alz.org /media/Documents/alzheimers-facts-and-figures.pdf.

What Is Alzheimer's Disease?

Alzheimer's disease is the most common cause of dementia, with up to four out of five cases of dementia being linked back to Alzheimer's disease. It is an irreversible, progressive brain disorder, the fifth leading cause of death in the US for adults age 65 and older, and it is estimated to affect more than 6.9 million Americans in 2024, including one in nine adults age 65 and older.[6] The number of new cases is expected to grow as the world population ages.

For most people with Alzheimer's disease, the first symptoms appear later in life, after age 65. Scientists don't yet fully understand what causes the disease, especially since it may be a result of complex brain changes that happen over decades. The National Institute on Aging suggests that probable causes include a combination of genetics, environment, and lifestyle. Less than 5 percent of cases are in adults 30 to 60 years of age, and those young-onset cases are most often related to family history, though some cases appear without any known cause.

Apolipoprotein E (APOE) genotyping is a genetic lab test that may help confirm a diagnosis of late-onset Alzheimer's disease in adults who show symptoms, but it cannot be the only tool used in diagnosis. If a person with dementia also has the APOE-e4 allele, it may be more likely that dementia is due to Alzheimer's disease, but it cannot prove it. In fact, there are no definitive diagnostic tests for Alzheimer's disease during life. This test is not appropriate for screening people without symptoms, and some people with APOE-e4 will never develop Alzheimer's disease.

Alzheimer's disease is commonly marked by memory loss, plus cognitive decline in one or more other areas, such as language skills, reasoning, attention, or visual perception. All cases of Alzheimer's

---

6 Alzheimer's Association, "2024 Alzheimer's Disease Facts and Figures."

disease involve cognitive decline, but not all cognitive decline is due to Alzheimer's disease.

Risk factors for late-onset Alzheimer's disease include:

- Older age
- Genetic factors (especially presence of APOE-e4)
- Family history
- History of head trauma
- Midlife high blood pressure (hypertension)
- Obesity
- Diabetes
- High cholesterol (hypercholesterolemia)

Alzheimer's Disease and Damage to the Brain

Some researchers hypothesize that oxidative stress and inflammation—which can come from eating unhealthy food, smoking, pollution, or illness—are at the root of Alzheimer's disease. Normally, the blood-brain barrier does a good job of protecting the brain. In early Alzheimer's disease, the blood-brain barrier begins to deteriorate, possibly due to chronic inflammation.

Imagine the healthy brain is a painter's canvas on which there are smooth, uniformly colored stars (neurons) connected by orderly lines, and only clean canvas in the background. Let's use this analogy to understand five changes going on in the brain with Alzheimer's disease.

1. There is a buildup of amyloid-beta protein (also called neuritic plaques) in between neurons, like messy splotches of unwanted paint marring the clean canvas.

2. Neurofibrillary tangles (twisted fibers that block nutrition from reaching all parts of the neuron) form inside neurons, as if someone added excess paint to the stars, creating a raised, uneven texture.

3. Neurons die off, as if someone washed away some of the stars on the canvas.

4. There's a loss of synapses, the gap between neurons required for them to communicate. The orderly lines between stars begin to disappear. Without synapses, neurons aren't very effective.

5. The brain tissue shrinks (also known as brain atrophy), eventually affecting nearly all of its functions, as if someone put the painter's canvas in the dryer so that the resulting canvas and everything on it is a lesser version of its original.

History of Alzheimer's Disease Discovery

Alzheimer's disease is named after Dr. Alois Alzheimer. In 1906, he had a patient who died of an unusual mental illness that caused her to suffer memory loss, have language problems, and engage in unpredictable behavior. After she died, he studied her brain tissue and found two types of abnormalities. Dr. Alzheimer found the abnormal clumps we now call plaques: amyloid plaques, beta-amyloid plaques, or amyloid-beta plaques. He also found tangled bundles of fibers in the neurons, which are now called neurofibrillary tangles, fibrillary tangles, or tau tangles.

How Mental Fitness Gets Tested

Mental fitness and its decline is measured based on five areas of brain functionality, through a variety of tests. The original MIND diet research used 19 standardized tests to evaluate the following five cognitive domains: episodic memory, semantic memory, perceptual speed, working memory, and visuospatial ability. Global cognition is measured in research studies by combining the results of a variety of tests measuring different cognitive domains to create a composite score.

Episodic memory is a three-step process involving the ability to register personal experiences of daily events and save them as memories that can be recalled later. Think of it as the memory that stores your individual view of the events of your life, much like what a forehead camera might capture in ongoing episodes in a television series called "my life." Examples of episodic memory include recalling where you parked your car this morning, the details of your wedding day, or remembering where you were and what you were doing when you found out about the 9/11 attacks in NYC.

The area of the brain important for this kind of memory is the medial temporal lobe (MTL). In the MIND diet research, it was evaluated based on results from a battery of seven tests, including: (1) word list memory, (2) word list recall, (3) word list recognition, (4) immediate recall of a story, (5) delayed recall of a story, and (6) immediate and (7) delayed recall of a second story.

Semantic memory is the brain's reserve of general knowledge and is the kind of memory that's very useful before an exam; it's all about facts and words. Unlike episodic memory, semantic memory isn't usually connected to a specific time or place. Examples of semantic memory are the general understanding of what a key is and how it works with a door, and remembering names of colors or state capitals. It even includes remembering what a cat is and understanding how to put a sentence together. These are tidbits of information that aren't necessarily linked to a personal experience. The difference between episodic memory and semantic memory is the difference between remembering what it was like when you met your best friend for the first time and recalling that you met on a certain date. The MIND diet research measured semantic memory through three tests: (1) a naming test, (2) a verbal fluency test, and (3) an abbreviated 15-item version of the National Adult Reading Test.

Perceptual speed is the ability to examine, compare, and contrast numbers, letters, and objects quickly. It was measured in the MIND diet research by four tests: (1) a symbol-digit test that asks for certain numbers to be matched with certain geometric shapes within a short period of time, such as 90 seconds, (2) a number comparison test to measure the ability to quickly and accurately compare numbers, (3) a 30-second test of how accurately a list of color names can be read out loud when the names of the colors are printed in mismatched colors (e.g., reading the word "blue" correctly even if it's printed in red ink), and (4) a 30-second test of naming the color of the ink when mismatched with a color's name (e.g., being able to say "red" while seeing the word "blue" written in red ink).

Working memory is a way to temporarily store information in order to complete a mental task. It can be thought of as a form of short-term memory. In other words, it's the ability to hold on to information long enough to use it right away. It's temporary storage of information for an express purpose. For example, working memory is what helps you dial a phone number someone has just read out loud to you, or to add 14 and 73 without using a calculator, pen and paper, or any other external tools. In the MIND diet research, it was measured by three tests: (1) digit span forward, (2) digit span backward, and (3) digit ordering tests. The first two tests determine memory span by measuring the longest list of items the tested person can recite back. The lists can be of numbers, letters, or words. For the MIND diet research, numbers were used. In the first memory span test (digit span forward), the test-taker had to recall the numbers in the order they were provided. In the second memory span test (digit span backward), the test-taker had to remember the numbers in the reverse order that they were provided; this is a more difficult test. In addition to these two memory span tests, the third test (digit ordering test) challenged working memory ability by asking the test-taker to memorize a set of numbers then recite them back in ascending order.

Visuospatial ability is the extent to which the brain can understand what it is seeing and process how it works. For example, this could include buttoning a shirt, putting together unassembled furniture, recognizing a triangle, or parking a car. It was measured by two tests: (1) a judgment of line orientation (JOLO) test, and (2) a standard progressive matrices (SPM) test. A JOLO test uses a semicircle with evenly distributed lines as the constant, then provides a series of lines in pairs. Both lines have to be accurately matched to one of the lines on the semicircle spectrum in order to pass.

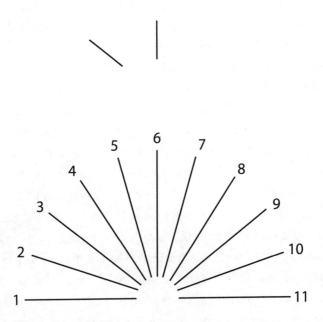

The second test, the SPM test, is a multiple-choice nonverbal test that asks the test-taker to complete a pattern or image with one of the provided options. The patterns get more difficult as the test goes on.

These 19 tests of the five cognitive domains are validated measures of cognitive function.

CHAPTER 2

THE MIND DIET STUDIES: HOW IT STARTED AND HOW IT'S GOING

What Is the MIND Diet?

The MIND diet is a healthy, evidence-based way to eat that is designed to help prevent Alzheimer's disease and delay cognitive decline. The original two MIND diet studies from 2015 show how the diet slows brain aging by 7.5 years and cuts the risk of developing Alzheimer's disease by 53 percent. The 150-plus research papers that have been published since then continue to show its benefits for cognition and more.

The MIND diet was developed by researchers from Rush University Medical Center and Harvard, led by Dr. Martha Clare Morris (1955 to 2020), to slow cognitive decline and reduce the risk of Alzheimer's disease. MIND is an acronym for Mediterranean-DASH diet intervention for neurodegenerative delay. As the acronym suggests, it is based on the Mediterranean and Dietary Approaches to Stop Hypertension (DASH) diets, but was then modified based on foods and nutrients shown to support brain health.

It consistently ranks highly in the annual *U.S. News & World Report's* "Best Diets Rankings." Top-ranked diets have to be easy to follow, nutritious, safe, effective for weight loss, and protective against diabetes and heart disease. The MIND diet does all that and hones in on the foods that specifically benefit brain health.

The MIND diet is a selection of the most brain-healthy foods from two well-established healthy diets, supported by what we currently know from nutrition and dementia research.

The MIND diet is made up of 15 components, including 10 brain-healthy food types to consume and five brain-harming ones to limit. The brain-healthy foods are leafy greens, more vegetables, berries, seafood, nuts, beans, whole grains, olive oil, lean poultry, and moderate intakes of wine. The brain-harming foods are butter and stick margarine, whole-fat cheese, fried fast foods, red meat, and pastries and sweets.

Earning the top MIND diet score of 15 means eating at least three servings of whole grains, one serving of vegetables, and one glass of wine each day; in addition, it means eating leafy greens nearly every day (at least six times a week), nuts most days of the week (at least five times a week), beans about every other day (four times a week), berries twice a week, lean poultry twice a week, fish once a week, and using olive oil as the main oil. Finally, it means limiting as much as possible the foods that aren't great for brain health, but definitely consuming less than one tablespoon of butter or margarine a day, pastries and sweets no more than four times a week, red meat no more than three times a week, whole-fat cheese no more than twice a month, and fried fast food no more than twice a month. Meeting each of these requirements earns one point each, adding up to a total possible score of 15.

It is worth noting that the MIND diet is less demanding than either the Mediterranean or DASH diets, with fewer required servings of fish, grains, fruits, and vegetables, and no emphasis on dairy or limits on total fat. The MIND diet is also different because it specifically recommends leafy greens and berries rather than fruits and vegetables in general.

The MIND diet's benefits to cognitive health make sense when considering the evidence-based approach to selecting its antioxidant-rich and anti-inflammatory foods, which protect the brain and make it harder for damaging plaques to form. Removing the brain-harming foods may be just as, if not more important, since eating too much of them contributes to chronic inflammation, damages the blood-brain barrier, and promotes the formation of beta-amyloid plaques.

MIND Diet Science: How It Started

One Smart Diet from Two Healthy Ones

Before there was a MIND diet, the Mediterranean and DASH diets were being studied for clues about how they affect cognitive decline, though that wasn't the focus. Since both diets have been shown to protect against high blood pressure, cardiovascular disease, stroke, and diabetes, looking at brain health was logical as those same conditions raise the risk for cognitive decline.

The Mediterranean diet is a plant-forward eating pattern that emphasizes fruits, vegetables, whole grains, beans, nuts, legumes, olive oil, herbs and spices, and seafood. In moderation, it also includes poultry, eggs, cheese, yogurt, and optional wine. It limits red meat and sweets. Research has proven its benefits for heart health and diabetes.

The DASH diet is also plant-forward. It is a clinical diet protocol that was designed to lower blood pressure and emphasizes grains, vegetables, fruit, low-fat or fat-free dairy, nuts, seeds, and legumes, with occasional lean meat, poultry, and fish. It limits fats, sweets, and salt. Rigorous studies show that following the DASH diet lowers blood pressure, increases beneficial HDL cholesterol, and decreases harmful LDL cholesterol and triglycerides.

The Mediterranean diet is different from the DASH diet in that olive oil is the main fat, there's a higher intake of fish, and it includes a moderate amount of wine with meals. The DASH diet is different from the Mediterranean diet in that it specifically restricts saturated fat and commercial pastries and sweets, and promotes dairy intake.

The MIND, Mediterranean, and DASH diets all share the idea of eating a foundation of natural, plant-based foods while limiting animal foods and foods high in saturated fat. The MIND diet is different in that it does not specifically recommend fruit, dairy, or multiple fish meals per week. It does, however, specifically recommend berries and leafy green vegetables.

Study 1: Cutting Alzheimer's Risk in Half

One of the first two MIND diet studies found that it's possible to reduce the risk of developing Alzheimer's disease by 35 to 53 percent by following the MIND diet. The results are from a multiyear study published in 2015 in *Alzheimer's & Dementia*, a top journal in the field. They show that the more closely the MIND diet was followed, the bigger the benefits. However, even moderately following it had a significant impact. Participant diets were also mapped against Mediterranean and DASH eating patterns for comparison. Overall, when it came to reducing Alzheimer's disease risk, the MIND diet performed best.

The study looked at data from 923 people aged 58 to 98 years, who volunteered to take part in Rush University's Memory and Aging Project (MAP). MAP data was used to compare how well their diets matched up with MIND, Mediterranean, and DASH diets, and how much that was associated with the development of Alzheimer's disease. The MAP population lived in retirement communities or senior public housing units in the Chicago area. They were tested at least twice to ensure they did not have Alzheimer's disease at the start of the study. Over the course of four and a half years of follow-up, 144 new cases of Alzheimer's disease were diagnosed.

When it came to seeing how much the participants' diets reflected the MIND, Mediterranean, and DASH diets, there was a wide range of results, from eating habits that looked a lot like these healthy diets to eating patterns that looked nothing like them. This is helpful because it means we can see how a spectrum of diets was associated with Alzheimer's disease. After all, if everyone in the study had very similar scores, it'd be hard to know if diet made a difference. These results were split into three groups, where the top scores were most closely aligned with the healthy diets.

For the MIND diet, study participants' diets were scored based on a total possible score of 15, one point for each of the 15 MIND diet components. The top third of scores averaged 9.6 on the 15-point MIND scale, with results ranging from 8.5 to 12.5. The middle third of scores averaged 7.5 points, ranging from 7 to 8 points. Both of these groups had a significantly lower risk of developing Alzheimer's disease. The top third cut their risk by 53 percent, and the middle third cut their risk by 35 percent. For the Mediterranean diet, the top third of scores had a protective effect, cutting risk by 54 percent. Similarly, it was the top third of scores for the DASH diet that was linked to a significant risk reduction, though it was lower at 39 percent.

The researchers considered why strictly following the DASH diet was not as protective as the other two diets. They looked at what was unique to the DASH diet—that is, a specific recommendation for dairy and low salt—and suggested that perhaps these guidelines may not be particularly important for brain health. What this all means is that following any of these diets strictly will have a benefit, but that the MIND diet brings brain health benefits even when halfway followed. Further, the MIND diet is less demanding in many ways, including fewer required servings of fish, grains, fruits, and vegetables, and no emphasis on dairy or limits on total fat.

It's tempting to wonder if the people with scores in the top third of the group were different in substantial ways. Maybe they were younger, more educated, exercised more, or took part in more brain-stimulating activities such as reading, playing games, writing letters, or visiting the library. However, the results controlled for all these factors and still found a statistically significant and clinically meaningful benefit to eating according to the MIND diet. The MIND diet was slightly less protective in people with the potential genetic marker for late-onset Alzheimer's disease, APOE-e4 (even though it's a marker, having it doesn't necessarily mean dementia is inevitable). It's important to note that the MIND diet was still protective in this group, just less so.

Another reasonable question to ask is if the results for the MIND diet were simply due to reducing the risk of diabetes, high blood pressure, stroke, and heart attack, which are all associated with an increased risk of Alzheimer's disease. While these factors certainly didn't hurt and were a natural benefit of a diet based on the Mediterranean and DASH diets, they were also controlled for, and the only difference was that the MIND diet was actually more brain-protective for people who had had a heart attack in the past. Overall, the effect of the MIND diet was independent of other healthy lifestyle choices or cardiovascular-related conditions.

The study's greatest strength is its robust methodology, including good design, sampling, data collection, and data analysis. Solid methods provide assurance that results are valid and credible.

A couple of notes about the population that was studied: First, the study participants were older adults, so it's hard to extend the findings to younger adults. However, the research does suggest that those who followed the diet longer were more protected against Alzheimer's, so it's reasonable to think there is a benefit to start following the MIND diet early. Second, the study population was mostly white, making it harder to definitively extend these findings to different ethnic or racial groups. That being said, the MIND diet is a generally healthy eating pattern based on two proven diets, and a safe and nutritious choice for most people, and we do now have data from other parts of the world (more on that soon).

Study 2: Slowing Cognitive Decline

The MIND diet can slow down brain aging by seven and a half years, according to another multiyear study published in 2015 in *Alzheimer's & Dementia*. Over nearly five years of follow-up, the MIND diet was shown to have a big impact on slowing the cognitive decline that comes with aging for adults whose average age was about 81 years. Similar to the study on diet and risk of Alzheimer's disease, the Mediterranean and DASH diets had brain-protective effects, but the strongest association was with the MIND diet.

The study looked at data from 960 people drawn from the more than 40 retirement communities and senior public housing units in the Chicago area that took part in Rush University's MAP. These people did not suffer from dementia at the beginning of the study and agreed to annual clinical neurological exams. However, out of 960 people, 220 had mild cognitive impairment to start. They were still included in the main analysis, though were taken out of additional secondary analysis. This is useful to see how the MIND diet can help those with mild symptoms of cognitive decline as well as those without any signs or symptoms of dementia yet. The MIND diet was found to be protective for the entire group, but even more so when the 220 were removed from the analysis, suggesting that eating for brain health before symptoms show up has bigger benefits.

The MIND diet scores for the group were divided into three tiers and compared to participant results from a battery of 19 cognitive tests that evaluated five cognitive domains: episodic memory, working memory, semantic memory, visuospatial ability, and perceptual speed. People in the top tier of MIND diet scores had higher scores across all five cognitive domains, with the strongest impact seen in three of the domains: episodic memory, semantic memory, and perceptual speed.

During the course of the study, 144 people dramatically improved or worsened how they ate. Since the dietary habits of these people changed over time, so did their MIND diet scores. To see if the inconsistent data from this portion of the group had much of an impact on the final results, the research team ran an analysis after removing this group. What they found was that doing so cleaned up the data, and the benefits of the MIND diet became even clearer and stronger. The global cognitive scores improved quite a bit as did most of the individual cognitive domains. These improved by 30 to 78 percent, with the exception of visuospatial ability, which remained stable.

To ensure these results were due to the MIND diet and not the cardiovascular protection provided by its foundation in the Mediterranean and DASH diets, the researchers controlled for high blood pressure, history of stroke or heart attack, and type 2 diabetes, but the results did not change. They also adjusted the results to account for differences in age, sex, education level, calorie intake, physical activity level, history of smoking, participation in cognitive activities, and even the genetic marker APOE-e4 that is more common in people with Alzheimer's disease. Still no appreciable effect on the beneficial results of the MIND diet. Last but not least, they took depression and obesity factors out of the picture, but adjusting for these factors also did not change any of the results. This all suggests that the MIND diet can indeed keep the brain cognitively younger despite a wide range of differences.

The study has additional strengths, including its up to 10 years of follow-up, annual evaluation of cognitive function using a series of standardized tests, and validated measuring tools to assess diet, controlling for confounding factors such as physical activity and education.

Preventing cognitive decline is more important than ever since it is an identifying characteristic of dementia. Delaying cognitive decline could mean delaying dementia by years. Even those not at risk for developing Alzheimer's dementia can benefit from slowing down the normal age-related downturn in cognitive abilities. Last but not least, the MIND diet has additional benefits for heart health, diabetes, and overall nutrition and well-being.

MIND Diet Science: How It's Going

Since the original MIND Diet studies were published in 2015, more than 150 additional scientific papers have been published. A little more than 60 percent of these studies are on memory, cognition, Alzheimer's disease, and dementia. The other 40 percent cover a variety of topics and populations from around the world. That said, the United States is where most of the research originates, followed by Europe, which combined make up about 70 percent of the papers. The most-researched topics among the other 40 percent of studies are cardiometabolic health, healthy aging, and mental health.

Aging increases the risk for many of these conditions. While we can't stop the passage of time, we can affect how we spend that time. Aging well is about maintaining independence and vitality so that we are able to live as many of our years as possible in good health. Some people call this our healthspan, in contrast to the lifespan. Unfortunately, chronic disease can rob us of good years. Healthy aging is about leaving no good years on the table. Eating nourishing foods is a fundamental piece of the answer, and research suggests the MIND diet is one way to get there.

Cognitive Health

Study 3: Follow-Up Trial of the MIND Diet

Reaching therapeutic levels of the MIND diet improved global cognition in a high-quality study led by many of the original MIND diet research team members at Rush University as well as a research team from Harvard University. This large, multi-site, three-year, randomized-controlled trial, whose findings were published in 2023, was a follow-up study to the original two observational studies from 2015.

The study included 604 older overweight adults around age 70 without dementia themselves, but who had a family history of dementia as well as a suboptimal diet. They were divided into either a MIND diet group that was provided with some of the key MIND diet foods (e.g., berries, nuts, olive oil), or a control group that focused on tracking calories, portion control, and strategies like goal-setting and mindful eating, but with the intention of keeping the types of foods the same. Instead of food, the control group regularly received $30 gift cards they could use for groceries, so they had a comparable amount of financial support to access food.

Both groups were coached on modest weight loss and were supported by dietitians throughout the three-year trial, with in-person counseling, group visits, phone consults, an online support group, and online food and weight tracking. For the first six months of the study, the dietitian-led counseling was weekly, followed by six months of contact every other week. For years two and three, participants were coached at least twice a month, and they always had the option to partake in individual and group sessions.

Here's what's interesting about the results. Both groups lost 5.5 percent body weight, which was above the target 3 to 5 percent. They reached this level of weight loss in six months and then maintained the weight loss for the rest of the three-year study. Many would call this a successful weight-loss trial, if nothing else, and the retention rate was very high. Nine in ten participants stuck with the study (93.4 percent) for the full three years. The only other randomized-controlled trial on the MIND diet supports this finding, though it was a small short-term three-month study. It found middle-aged women (~48 years old) who followed the MIND diet versus their usual diet (the control) lost more weight and had lower body fat percentages and waist circumferences, even though both groups were counseled to eat fewer calories overall.

Even more interesting for brain health and overall well-being, both groups improved their diet scores on a 14-point MIND scale (it wasn't the original 15-point scale because wine was removed from the clinical trial for safety reasons). Both groups started at a moderate 7.7 score and ended with an impressive 11.1 score (MIND diet group) and a still good 8.5 (control group). Recall that in the earlier MIND diet studies, the top scores that were the most protective against cognitive decline and risk of Alzheimer's disease were in the 8.5 to 12.5 range. So the control group's diet didn't improve as much as the MIND diet group, which is to be expected, but it still improved enough to reach the bottom of the therapeutic range. This was good for the control group's personal health, but it also meant that the "control" group didn't really provide a control diet to compare to since it didn't stay stable.

Therefore, technically, this study didn't prove the MIND diet improved cognition any more than a control diet. Upon closer inspection, we see that both groups improved their diet into the therapeutic range (8.5 to 12.5) seen in the original observational studies. This may explain why both groups improved their cognitive performance. However, more research is needed to confirm this hypothesis.

In the meantime, what does the rest of the research say about the MIND diet and brain health? There are nearly a hundred papers exploring this topic. Of those, the highest quality studies point in a positive direction. They all suggest following the MIND diet is linked to better global cognition and a reduced risk of Alzheimer's disease. There's good evidence that the MIND diet is associated with better episodic memory and a reduced risk of all dementias too. We have less research on mild cognitive impairment, subjective memory complaints, and cognitive resilience, but so far the results are promising. Last but not least, we don't yet have enough research on the MIND diet's influence on cognitive decline over time, nor about the effect the MIND diet has on signs of brain health such as brain volume (we don't want too much shrinkage), or amyloid plaques or tau tangles, which are abnormal clusters of proteins that can accumulate in the brain and are considered to be hallmarks of Alzheimer's disease. So far, the few studies exploring these topics have come back with either positive or neutral results. Overall, the outlook is positive, but more research is needed.

Heart Health

Have you heard that heart health is brain health? Research studies on the Mediterranean and DASH diets showed us that diets well-known for being heart-healthy also slowed cognitive decline. That makes sense because the brain relies on a healthy heart. The brain is highly vascularized, with a vast network of blood vessels. The heart pumps 20 to 25 percent of the body's blood to the head, carrying with it vital nutrients for brain health and fueling it with one in every five calories we eat. So, heart-healthy eating is the foundation for fueling brain health. But is brain health heart health?

The answer is yes, according to several studies, including those that incorporate large and nationally representative data from the United States. In two studies from 2023 that delved into the

National Health and Nutrition Examination Survey data, people with atherosclerosis or stroke lived longer if they followed most of the MIND diet guidelines (scores of 8.5 and up). They were also 24 percent less likely to have high blood pressure and 29 percent less likely to have atherosclerotic cardiovascular disease.[7] In another study, people with higher MIND diet scores had healthier hearts, which was measured by better left ventricular function. The left ventricle of the heart works harder than any of the other heart chambers. It's important because it pumps oxygenated blood to the body, so failure here negatively impacts all organs. This was in a 2021 study of 2,512 adults from the Framingham Heart Study, one of the US's largest and longest running population-based studies of factors contributing to cardiovascular and other diseases.[8]

Diabetes

Alzheimer's disease has been called "type 3 diabetes" by researchers for the past 20 years, though it's not an officially diagnosed type of diabetes. A 2020 paper in the *Lancet Journal of Neurology* reviews the critical role of insulin in brain health, and how insulin resistance in the brain can contribute to brain aging, cognitive impairment, and Alzheimer's disease. There is more to learn in this area, but we know people with type 2 diabetes are at a higher risk of developing Alzheimer's disease, and that a healthy diet helps manage diabetes. Recent research on the MIND diet supports this idea.

In a large study of more than 6,800 people, those with diabetes who closely followed the MIND diet had a better chance of living

---

7 Song et al., "The Value of the MIND Diet in the Primary and Secondary Prevention of Hypertension," *Frontiers in Nutrition* 10 (2023): 1129667, https://doi.org/10.3389/fnut.2023.1129667.

8 M. E. Walker et al., "Associations of the Mediterranean-Dietary Approaches to Stop Hypertension Intervention for Neurodegenerative Delay Diet with Cardiac Remodelling in the Community: The Framingham Heart Study," *British Journal of Nutrition* 126, no. 12 (2021): 1888–1896, https://doi.org/10.1017/S0007114521000660.

longer compared to those who didn't follow it as closely.[9] The study, which included more than 1,000 people with diabetes, showed people with diabetes who had higher MIND diet scores (8 to 13) were 25 percent less likely to die from any cause and 50 percent less likely to die from cardiovascular disease. For what it's worth, people without diabetes who followed the MIND diet also enjoyed a 17 percent reduced risk of dying from any cause.

In a separate large study of 8,750 adults, different approaches to evaluating diet quality were compared to rates of diabetes.[10] Better adherence to the MIND diet and lower dietary inflammatory scores (DIS) stood out as they were associated with the lowest rates of diabetes. The DIS is a relatively recent dietary scoring system used in research to rates foods based on the inflammatory markers they create when eaten. Higher scores are more inflammatory, so lower scores are more desirable. The other standards against which diets were measured were the Mediterranean diet, DASH diet, plant-based, Southern US, and dietary inflammatory index, which is similar to DIS, except it measures dietary contribution to inflammation based on nutrients instead of food.

Metabolic Syndrome

One in three adults in the US have metabolic syndrome, also called insulin resistance syndrome. It's a group of conditions that together raise the risk of cognitive impairment and dementia as well as heart disease, diabetes, and stroke. Someone has metabolic syndrome when they have three or more of the following five risk factors: a large waistline, high blood pressure, high blood sugar, high blood triglycerides (which can raise the levels of harmful LDL cholesterol), or low HDL cholesterol ("good" cholesterol that helps remove LDL).

9 Song et al., "Association between MIND Diet Adherence and Mortality," *Nutrition & Diabetes* 13, no. 1 (2023): 18, https://doi.org/10.1038/s41387-023-00247-1.

10 Tison et al., "Differences in the Association of Select Dietary Measures with Risk of Incident Type 2 Diabetes," *Diabetes Care* 45, no. 11 (2022).

The good news is that it is preventable, and research suggests the MIND diet can help. In a 2023 study, only adults with higher MIND diet scores had less visceral fat (often called belly fat) and better levels of all metabolic syndrome risk factors compared to people following Mediterranean, DASH, or the *Dietary Guidelines for Americans 2020–2025*, which were associated with improvements in some but not all risk factors, and none of the other diets were associated with reduced belly fat.[11]

Mental Health

Given that the same organ is central to both cognitive and mental health, it's no wonder researchers were curious to learn if the MIND diet could help with some of the most common mental health concerns such as stress, anxiety, and depression. While this is a newer area of study, the majority of the research in this area shows that people who follow the MIND diet well are less likely to suffer from depression. The data on anxiety and stress is more mixed, with results being either positive or neutral. For example, a 2023 study found that people with very high MIND scores (9.5 to 13) were 97 percent less likely to have anxiety disorders, especially as the diet quality went up.[12] A 2022 study found that people with the highest MIND scores, out of four groupings, were 39 percent less likely to have anxiety.[13] But a 2019 study found being better at following the MIND diet

11 Holthaus et al., "MIND Dietary Pattern Adherence Is Inversely Associated with Visceral Adiposity and Features of Metabolic Syndrome," *Nutrition Research* 116 (2023): 69–79, https://doi.org/10.1016/j.nutres.2023.06.001.

12 K. Torabynasab et al., "Adherence to the MIND Diet Is Inversely Associated with Odds and Severity of Anxiety Disorders," *BMC Psychiatry* 23, no. 1 (2023): 330, https://doi.org/10.1186/s12888-023-04776-y.

13 R. Barkhordari et al., "The Relation between MIND Diet with Psychological Disorders and Psychological Stress among Iranian Adults," *BMC Psychiatry* 22, no. 1 (2022): 496, https://doi.org/10.1186/s12888-022-04128-2.

recommendations was associated with less stress, but not anxiety.[14] These are all observational studies.

In a unique 2022 four-week pilot study among older Chinese adults, following the MIND diet along with spending time in nature (forest bathing) reduced anxiety and negative mood states compared to the MIND diet alone.[15] Total cholesterol, LDL cholesterol, triglycerides, and glucose levels were also all significantly lower. Indeed, in other studies, physical activity has been shown to enhance the brain health benefits of the MIND diet. In this study, participants spent two hours each weekend (four sessions total) immersed in a guided group experience through nature with a mix of leisurely walking, sitting, and standing while being invited to use their senses to enjoy the moment, slow down physically and mentally, and build connections to the forest. They rested and shared their experiences within the group between each activity. Each session ended with a tea ceremony. Pilot studies are meant to inspire larger, more robust studies, but in the meantime, this adds to the evidence that nutrition and nature (and perhaps movement and connections with others) may work together to promote better mental health.

Parkinson's Disease and Parkinsonism

Parkinson's disease, like Alzheimer's disease, is a neurodegenerative disease that affects older adults, and for which there is no cure. It is the most common, but not only, cause of parkinsonism, which refers to neurological disorders with similar symptoms such as tremors, muscle rigidity, poor balance, and slow movement. A person with

---

14 A. Salari-Moghaddam et al., "Adherence to the MIND Diet and Prevalence of Psychological Disorders in Adults," *Journal of Affective Disorders* 256 (2019): 96–102, https://doi.org/10.1016/j.jad.2019.05.056.

15 K.-Y. Yau et al., "Cardiac and Mental Benefits of Mediterranean-DASH Intervention for Neurodegenerative Delay (MIND) Diet Plus Forest Bathing (FB) versus MIND Diet among Older Chinese Adults: A Randomized Controlled Pilot Study," *International Journal of Environmental Research and Public Health* 19, no. 22 (2022): 14665, https://doi.org/10.3390/ijerph192214665.

parkinsonism may also have non-movement related symptoms such as changes to mood, thinking, sleep, and speech. Just as Alzheimer's disease is the most common cause of dementia, Parkinson's is the most common cause of parkinsonism.

A recent study found that people following the MIND diet were less likely to develop parkinsonism.[16] The same study found that in people who already had parkinsonism, following the MIND diet was associated with a slower progression of the disease. Older adults with an average MIND score of 10 (out of 15) had a 42 percent reduced risk of parkinsonism, and those with an average MIND score of 8 had a 30 percent reduced risk. This was compared to 706 older adults (who were on average 80 years of age at the start of the study) followed for an average of 4.6 years, with an average MIND score of 6.5. This study also looked at the Mediterranean diet and DASH diet. Those with the highest Mediterranean diet scores reduced their risk of developing parkinsonism by a modest 3 percent and slowed the progression of the condition. The DASH diet had no benefit for reducing the risk of developing parkinsonism or the severity of the disease. The researchers hypothesized that the MIND diet's specifically brain-healthy foods may be responsible for its stronger benefits for motor and cognitive function. They noted that leafy greens and berries are two of its unique components.

The MIND diet was shown to be twice as effective as the Mediterranean diet in reducing the severity of Parkinson's disease symptoms, according to a 2022 observational study of 1,205 adults ages 36 to 90 living with Parkinson's. Another study[17] compared the diets of 167 participants with Parkinson's disease to 119 control participants and found that women following the MIND diet delayed

16   P. Agarwal et al., "MIND Diet Associated with Reduced Incidence and Delayed Progression of Parkinsonism in Old Age," *Journal of Nutrional Health and Aging*, 22 (2018): 1211–1215, doi: 10.1007/s12603-018-1094-5.

17   A. Metcalfe-Roach et al., "MIND and Mediterranean Diets Associated with Later Onset of Parkinson's Disease," *Movement Disorders* 36, no. 4 (2021): 977–984, doi: 10.1002/mds.28464.

the onset of Parkinson's by up to 17.4 years compared to those with a low MIND diet score. Following a Mediterranean diet was also associated with a later onset of Parkinson's, especially in men who delayed onset by up to 8.4 years. Regardless of which dietary pattern people followed, the most protective foods were vegetables, nuts, beans, and fruit. The best foods to limit were butter, margarine, cheese, fried fast food, pastries and sweets, red meat, and soda.

Healthy Aging

If we are fortunate, we live long lives. Of course, getting older comes with its challenges. Recent research suggests the MIND diet may help with common age-related issues.

Following the MIND diet was associated with better muscle strength, slower physical decline, and lower odds of physical functional impairment (measured by repeated chair stands, standing balance, and gait speed), according to a 2022 study by Talegawkar et al. In this observational study, adults ages 30 to 101 in the Baltimore area were followed for an average of 6 years and grouped by how well they followed the MIND diet. Out of a possible 15, the bottom tertile had MIND scores of 3.5 to 7.8, the second tertile had scores of 7.8 to 9.3, and the top tertile had scores of 9.3 to 13. For adults ages 60 and older, the top tertile saw 57 percent lower odds of physical functional impairment, slower physical decline, and better grip strength compared to the bottom group. Often we only see a benefit when there is something wrong to start with, but in this study even adults with good physical functionality and grip strength to start had lower odds of physical functional impairment over time.

In another study, MIND diet followers in the Chicago area were able to live more independently than those who followed the Mediterranean or DASH diets.[18] This study included adults ages 58

---

18 Agarwal et al., "Dietary Patterns and Self-Reported Incident Disability in Older Adults," *The Journals of Gerontology* 74, no. 8 (2019): 1331–1337, https://doi.org/10.1093/gerona/gly211.

to 97 and measured three things. One, 809 adults were studied for how well participants performed activities of daily living (ADL), which includes feeding, bathing, dressing, going to the bathroom, transferring (e.g., getting in and out of bed, going from sitting to standing), and walking across a small room. Two, it measured instrumental activities of daily living (IADL) in 471 adults, which includes how well participants independently used telephones, prepared meals, managed money, managed medications, took care of light and heavy housekeeping, shopped, and traveled within a local area. Three, it measured mobility among 551 adults, including how independently participants walked up and down a flight of stairs, walked a half mile, and did heavy housework.

Again, the study population was divided into three groups by MIND diet score. The bottom group had an average MIND score of 6.5 (range was 3 to 7), the middle group's average score was 8 (range was 7.5 to 8.5), and the top group's average was 10 (range was 9 to 13). All scores were out of a possible 15. Top followers of the MIND diet had 33 percent lower rates of ADL disability compared to the bottom group. The middle group also had lower rates of ADL disability (25 percent) compared to the bottom group. In comparison, only the top followers of the Mediterranean diet (27 percent lower rates) and DASH (25 percent lower rates) saw benefits.

For IADL disability, only the MIND diet continued to show benefits, reducing the risk by 21 percent for the top group and 20 percent for the middle group. Since IADL involves cognitive functions, the researchers suggest that the MIND diet's effect on cognition translated to better IADL performance. Finally, all three dietary patterns were associated with better mobility. The top two MIND diet groups reduced the risk of impaired mobility by 27 percent and 22 percent, compared to only the top Mediterranean and DASH groups, which reduced the risk of impaired mobility by 22 percent and 27 percent. Overall, people who followed about half (53 percent) to two-thirds (67 percent) of the MIND diet recommendations saw benefits for ADL, IADL, and mobility, which means it may be a simpler approach to support healthy aging than the Mediterranean or DASH diets.

A large long-term study in Hong Kong provides support for the idea that the MIND diet helps the aging brain (and body) because it is anti-inflammatory.[19] This study was in 2,802 older men and women who were followed for 14 years. It found that people with higher MIND diet scores had lower blood markers of inflammaging, and had a 37 percent reduced risk of dying from cardiovascular disease. Inflammaging refers to an age-related rise in pro-inflammatory substances in the blood and tissues that increase the risk for several diseases and disability in older adults.

Premature Death

The study of mortality is about understanding what helps us live longer in better health versus what prematurely cuts our lives short. Recent research suggests that following the MIND diet is associated with a longer life expectancy, with lower odds of premature death from type 2 diabetes or atherosclerotic cardiovascular disease, and with more years lived without Alzheimer's disease.

In a 2022 study, the MIND diet was a component of a healthy lifestyle that was associated with more years lived overall, with more of those years in good health.[20] Participants had a longer life expectancy with more remaining years lived without Alzheimer's disease. This is according to a study in 2,449 men and women aged 65

---

19 Chan et al., "How Dietary Patterns Are Related to Inflammaging and Mortality in Community-Dwelling Older Chinese Adults in Hong Kong—A Prospective Analysis," *The Journal of Nutrition, Health & Aging* 23, no. 2 (2019): 181–194, https://doi.org/10.1007/s12603-018-1143-0.

20 K. Dhana et al., "Healthy Lifestyle and Life Expectancy with and without Alzheimer's Dementia," *British Medical Journal* 377, no. e068390 (2022), https://doi.org/10.1136/bmj-2021-068390.

years and older in the Chicago area. Five healthy lifestyle factors were measured, including following the MIND diet, late-life cognitive activities, moderate to vigorous activity, no smoking, and light to moderate alcohol intake. People who regularly took part in four to five of these behaviors benefitted the most compared to those who only engaged in zero to one activity. This is more support for the argument that a healthy diet is essential for well-being, and that the benefits are only enhanced by combining with other healthy lifestyle habits.

Two 2023 studies by Song et al. using data from the nationally representative National Health and Nutrition Examination Survey (NHANES) in the US found that patients with atherosclerotic cardiovascular disease (ASCVD), stroke, or type 2 diabetes were less likely to die prematurely in general, but especially from cardiovascular disease. In one of the studies, 943 adults with ASCVD or stroke lowered their risk of premature death by 10 percent for every one point increase in MIND diet score. The risk of death from cardiovascular disease was even lower: 16 percent reduced risk per point increase in MIND diet score. The top group had scores of 8.5 or above, the middle group had scores of 7.5 to 8, and the bottom group had scores of 7 or below. The top and middle groups both reduced their risk. Compared to the bottom group, the top group reduced their risk of premature death by nearly half (48 percent).

In the second study, among 1,021 patients with type 2 diabetes, those who had MIND diet scores above 8 reduced their risk of premature death by 25 percent and their risk of cardiovascular death by 50 percent compared to those who had scores of 8 or below. This was part of a larger study of 6,887 adults, and those without diabetes also benefited. A high MIND diet score reduced the risk of premature death from any cause by 17 percent.

Adapting the MIND Diet to Cultures Outside the US

Early evidence shows promising results for adapting the MIND diet to other cultures. There are both cultural and clinical reasons to respect heritage foods and dietary practices. First and foremost, food and culture are so closely tied together that any dietary guidance must respect and honor cultural heritage in order to support whole-person well-being. This kind of approach offers choice, dignity, respect, self-determination, and purposeful living. Clinically, dietary advice that fits into cultural norms are more likely to be accepted and followed, which means it's realistic and sustainable, which leads to better outcomes.

Observational research has shown that the MIND diet works better in North America, and the Mediterranean diet and Nordic diets work better in those regions. For example, there are positive findings for the MIND diet from around the world, but most of the strongest come from the United States. The Mediterranean diet is associated with a lower risk of mortality in several countries, but the effect is stronger in Mediterranean nations. The best diet for brain health in a Swedish population seems to be a Nordic one. How can this be? Researchers point to differences in cultural practices between populations.

For example, in one culture red meat may be consumed in lean forms and in smaller portion sizes compared to larger portions of vegetables and whole grains, while in another culture, red meat may be primarily consumed in large burgers on white-flour buns, with a side of fried foods and sugary soda. In another example, berries are a MIND-specific food that are part of some but not all cultures. In both of these examples, the MIND scoring system might capture different dietary patterns depending on cultural practices. This means that, although the MIND diet is a sound approach to brain health and overall well-being, people will have the best success with it if they thoughtfully adapt it to their own cultural foods and traditions. Some research bears this out.

For example, in a French study, berries were replaced by total polyphenol intake; in a Chinese population, wine was replaced with green tea; and in a Korean study, olive oil was replaced by perilla oil, which is made from perilla seeds and is rich in plant-based omega-3s. There were additional changes, but these are a few key examples. The 2022 French study found that the French MIND diet was associated with a reduced risk of dementia and preservation of the brain's white matter.[21] The two studies in China used an adapted MIND diet called China MIND, or cMIND. In studies from 2022 and 2024, higher cMIND scores were associated with a reduced risk of cognitive impairment, better cognitive function, and greater ease with IADL.[22] In a small 12-week clinical study in a Korean population, women aged 60 and older who followed the Korean MIND diet, or K-MIND diet, saw improvements in cognitive function.[23] This study also measured biomarkers and found that the K-MIND diet enhanced energy production, suppressed molecules that lead to inflammation, and supported systems that help produce neurotransmitters and maintain brain cell membranes.

21 A. Thomas et al., "Association of a MIND Diet with Brain Structure and Dementia in a French Population," *Journal of Prevention of Alzheimer's Disease* 9, no. 4 (2022): 655–664. doi: 10.14283/jpad.2022.67.

22 X. Huang et al., "Development of the cMIND Diet and Its Association with Cognitive Impairment in Older Chinese People," *Journal of Nutrition, Health & Aging* 26, no. 8 (2022): 760–770, https://doi.org/10.1007/s12603-022-1829-1; W. Lin et al., "Association of Adherence to the Chinese Version of the MIND Diet with Reduced Cognitive Decline in Older Chinese Individuals, *Journal of Nutrition, Health & Aging* 28, no. 2 (2024): 100024, https://doi.org/10.1016/j.jnha.2023.100024.

23 E. Y. Kang et al., "Modified Korean MIND Diet: A Nutritional Intervention for Improved Cognitive Function in Elderly Women through Mitochondrial Respiration, Inflammation Suppression, and Amino Acid Metabolism Regulation," *Molecular Nutrition & Food Research* 67, no. 20 (2023): 2300329, https://doi.org/10.1002/mnfr.202300329.

Though these studies were conducted in populations outside the US, they provide insight into how the MIND diet may be adapted to dietary traditions practiced by the increasingly diverse population within the US, and therefore better serve all communities.

THE MIND DIET IN KOREA AND CHINA

Separately, researchers in Korea and China adapted the MIND diet to their cultural foods, respectively, and found associations with better cognitive function. Here's a quick look at the adapted MIND diet guidelines used in research in Korea and China.

Korean MIND Diet[24]

- Vegetables, 6x/week
- Nuts, 6x/week
- Whole grains, 6x/week
- Perilla oil or powder, 6x/week
- Milk or fermented milk, 6x/week
- Water, 6x/week
- Legumes, 3x/week
- Fruits, 3x/week
- Berries, 3x/week
- Tomatoes, 3x/week
- Fish, 1x/week
- Poultry, 1x/week
- Social interaction, 1x/week 30+ min
- Physical activity, 1x/week 30+min
- No alcohol

---

24   Kang et al., "Modified Korean MIND Diet."

Chinese MIND Diet[25]

- Whole grains, 250-400g/d
- Fresh vegetables, 6x/week
- Mushroom or algae, 4x/week
- Fresh fruit, 6x/week
- Vegetable oil
- Fish, 1x/week
- Soybeans, 4x/week
- Nuts
- Garlic, 4x/week
- Green tea, ~daily
- Pastries/sweets < 1x/month

What's In Store

Researchers are actively studying the MIND diet. There are very early findings (sometimes only one study) on some topics that we may come to learn more about in the future. For now, there are very early positive or neutral findings about the MIND diet's effects on breast cancer risk, children's attention span, glaucoma risk, glioma risk, odds of developing irritable bowel syndrome, severity and length of migraine, multiple sclerosis risk, and sleep quality. Stay tuned.

---

25 Huang et al., "Development of the MIND Diet"; Wenjian Lin, Xiaoyu Zhou, and Xueyuan, "Association of Adherence to the Chinese Version of the MIND Diet," *The Journal of Nutrition, Health and Aging* 28, no.2 (2024), https://doi.org/10.1016/j.jnha.2023.100024.

CHAPTER 3
BRAIN-HEALTHY FOODS

Vegetables

Vegetables, leafy greens in particular, are emphasized in the MIND diet. Past population-based studies have reported that people who best maintained their cognitive abilities ate more vegetables, especially green, leafy vegetables. Green, leafy vegetables provide folate, vitamin E, carotenoids, and flavonoids, which have been related to a lower risk of dementia and cognitive decline in lab settings too.

To test the connection, researchers from Brigham and Women's Hospital and Harvard School of Public Health started looking at vegetables (and fruit) as possible protectors of cognitive health. They reduce the risk of cardiovascular disease, and cardiovascular disease is linked to an increased risk of cognitive decline. The researchers studied more than a decade's worth of diet records from 13,000 older women in search of links to cognitive performance, cognitive decline, and episodic memory in particular, since this type of memory is one of the stronger predictors for Alzheimer's disease.

A serving of vegetables per day protected against cognitive decline, equal to being about one and a half years younger, cognitively speaking. Of the vegetables, the strongest protective effect was seen for green, leafy vegetables such as spinach or romaine. On average, people ate anywhere from one-third of a serving to about a serving and a half with greater benefits for higher intakes. A serving of fresh leafy greens is a cup; for cooked greens, a serving is half a cup.

A 2018 study of older adults confirmed that leafy greens, especially those in the cabbage family, such as kale and bok choy, are among the best vegetables for brain health. With one to two servings per day, participants slowed their brain aging by 11 years compared to those who rarely or never ate leafy greens.[26]

Cruciferous vegetables such as broccoli and cauliflower were also clear winners for cognitive performance. The group who ate the most cruciferous vegetables, out of five groups, performed better at cognitive tests, especially for episodic memory. Compared to the lowest intake group (who ate less than 2 tablespoons of cruciferous vegetables a day), those in the highest intake group (who ate closer to a Half cup serving per day) performed at a level equivalent to being almost two years cognitively younger. The benefits to cognitive aging started showing up at the fourth highest intake group out of five (eating between about a quarter cup and a half cup of cruciferous vegetables a day). Therefore, there may be a cognitive health-related benefit to making one of your servings of daily vegetables a cruciferous one.

The researchers note that folate might be an important nutrient that may help explain the positive results for vegetables in general, as well as leafy greens and cruciferous vegetables in particular. Folate intake has been associated with cognitive function and dementia in other population-based studies. There's also a reasonable rationale for how it works. Without enough folate, levels of homocysteine can rise too high. In cell and animal studies, high homocysteine levels are toxic to neurons. Folate is found naturally in many wholesome foods, including dark green, leafy vegetables, citrus fruits, legumes, and

---

26 M. Morris et al., "Nutrients and Bioactives in Green Leafy Vegetables and Cognitive Decline," *Neurology* 90, no. 3 (2018): e214–e222, https://doi.org/10.1212/WNL.000000000 0004815.

vegetables in general. Though it's found in both fruits and vegetables, overall, vegetables are a better source of this important nutrient.

In addition to folate, additional key bioactive nutrients in leafy green vegetables are phylloquinone (vitamin K) and the carotenoid lutein. Each of these have been independently associated with slowing down cognitive decline. The more of these nutrients people consumed, the better their brain health was. Morris et al. discuss how a three-year randomized trial in people known to have low folic acid levels found that supplementation with folic acid slowed down cognitive decline. Phylloquinone hasn't been extensively studied, but Morris discusses one study finding that better phylloquinone intake was related to better scores on the Mini-Mental State Examination, a screening tool that evaluates multiple aspects of cognition and can be used repeatedly over time to monitor cognitive function and detect cognitive impairment. Good levels of lutein, a carotenoid also found in egg yolks, was associated with a reduced risk of dementia. A small study in adults in their eighties and hundreds found that the more lutein there was in the brain and blood, the higher cognitive scores were. Lutein in particular preferentially builds up in the brain and eyes, and is the only carotenoid that is allowed to cross the blood-brain barrier along with its close cousin zeaxanthin (they're often found together in foods).

The MIND diet includes a daily serving of any vegetable, plus a near-daily serving of leafy greens per week (six servings a week). To make it simple, consider adopting a daily green salad habit.

Some of the most commonly eaten vegetables in the United States are potatoes (much of it as fries or chips), lettuce, onions, tomatoes (much of it as pasta sauce), carrots, corn, green beans, peppers, and broccoli. These are great, but there is so much more to the vegetable world.

Generally, for quality and food safety, buy vegetables that are not bruised, slimy, or otherwise damaged. When buying precut veggies, make sure they come from a refrigerated area; if it's not refrigerated, it should be surrounded by ice. Fresh veggies should be kept separate from raw meat, poultry, and seafood in the cart, at checkout, and at home. For the convenience minded, packaged salad greens are available in prewashed ready-to-eat packages. However, adding a handling step means another opportunity to introduce food safety risks and will usually come at a premium cost, so only buy from growers or brands you trust. Frozen and canned vegetables are another healthy and nutritious option available all year round.

There are so many vegetables to enjoy, and that variety is part of their nutritional charm. By eating a rainbow of vegetables, the brain (and body) benefit from a greater range of nutrients it can use to thrive. This list scratches the surface. A local farmer's market, your local grocer, or specialty markets (e.g., Korean market like H-Mart, Mexican market Northgate) may expose you to additional produce to try.

Year-Round Leafy Greens

Leafy greens hit their stride in the spring, but various greens are available in other seasons, and some are available year round. A few tips: The best way to wash leafy greens (unless it's labeled as prewashed) is to agitate them in a large bowl of water so any dirt and debris sinks to the bottom, then lift them out of the water into another bowl. Sometimes, it takes a couple rounds to get them clean. If you have wilted greens, they can often be brought back to life by soaking them in ice water for 10 minutes or more, which shocks them into accepting water into their cells, helping them to regain some crispness. The extent to which this will work may depend on how far gone your greens are, but before tossing wilted greens, it's worth giving this method a try. Or, use wilted greens as-is in soups, stir-fries, and smoothies.

Amaranth—not to be confused with the whole grain by the same name, this refers to the amaranth plant's leaves, not the seeds (grains).

A beautiful leafy green with reddish veins, amaranth is also known as Chinese spinach, with a flavor between spinach and mild cabbage. Its stems can be prepared like asparagus, and the leaves can be treated like spinach. Choose crisp bunches with no signs of insect damage. It can be stored in a plastic bag in the refrigerator for up to a week. Amaranth is rich in vitamins A, C, and K. It provides calcium, and can be added to salads and soups alike.

Bok choy—a delicate leafy green that lends itself well to a quick steam or sauté (especially baby bok choy, which is milder than its adult version), bok choy has been grown in China for more than 6,000 years. It can also be eaten fresh. Alternate names are pak choi, bok choi, and Chinese cabbage. It's an excellent source of vitamins A and C, and a good source of folate. Look for firm stalks and fresh-looking, unwilted leaves without brown spots. Store in a plastic bag for up to a week, unwashed.

Cabbage—an affordable superfood that is high in vitamin C and low in calories, green cabbage stays fresh when refrigerated for up to a week. Keep in mind that vitamin C is destroyed through heated cooking, so a raw marinated slaw will save more of its nutrition. Look for cabbage heads that feel heavy for their size, with tight leaves.

Dandelion greens—dandelions are technically weeds, but value is in the eye of the beholder. The greens are packed with vitamins A, C, and K, fiber, calcium, manganese, iron, and B vitamins B1, B2, and B6. The small, jagged leaves are bitter with a peppery flavor, similar to arugula. They can be used raw in a salad, tossed with a citrus vinaigrette that's vibrant enough to stand up to the bitter notes. Dandelion greens also work great mixed into soups, warm grain salads, and braised on their own.

Gai lan—sometimes called Chinese kale or Chinese broccoli, gai lan is a dark green leafy vegetable with smoother, more tender leaves than either kale or broccoli. It's easy to enjoy this vegetable steamed or sautéed. Gai lan is an excellent source of vitamins A and C, and also provides a good source of iron and calcium. Look for fresh stalks and dark green leaves without any brown spots. Store unwashed in a plastic bag in the refrigerator for up to three days.

Salad Savoy(R)—this bright purple and green leafy vegetable is a child of the 1980s, developed by John Moore and grown in Salinas, California. It's an excellent source of vitamins A, C, and fiber. Look for vibrantly colored leaves and avoid any limp or yellowing leaves. It can be stored for up to five days, unwashed, in the refrigerator, wrapped in a damp paper towel and paper bag.

Swiss chard—the leaves resemble flat kale, and its stem resembles celery. The stems can be green, red, or a rainbow mix of reds, pinks, oranges, and yellows. A hearty vegetable, Swiss chard can be used in soups, scrambles, quiche, and stir fry, or steamed. With all the varieties, some sort of Swiss chard is always in season. It's an excellent source of vitamins A and C, and also provides magnesium. Look for fresh green leaves and avoid discolored or yellowing leaves. It can be stored unwashed in plastic bags in the refrigerator crisper for two to three days.

Fall Greens

Butter lettuce—see Spring.
  Endive—see Summer.
  Ong choy spinach—see Summer.

Winter Greens

Kale—a member of the cabbage family, kale is an excellent source of vitamins A and C, and also provides calcium and potassium. There are several varieties of kale, from the common curly kale to the smoother (but still bumpy) and darker lacinato kale, also known as dinosaur kale. Kale can be stored in a plastic bag in the coldest part of the refrigerator (the bottom, back) for up to five days. Though it is a winter vegetable, its popularity has made it a year-round staple at many grocery stores.

Spring Greens

Butter lettuce—this mild, slightly sweet, and buttery lettuce is an excellent source of vitamin A, and a good source of vitamin C and folate. Boston lettuce and Bibb lettuce are both types of butter lettuce. Look for fresh-looking leaves without signs of wilting. It can be washed, dried, and stored in a plastic bag for up to five days in the refrigerator. Sometimes butter lettuce is sold as "living lettuce" with roots still attached to dirt in order to preserve freshness. For this kind of butter lettuce, store it as-is, remove the roots, and rinse just before using.

Collard greens—part of the cabbage family, collard greens grow in a loose bouquet and can be cooked quickly, but also stand up to slow-cooking methods like stewing and braising. These greens are an excellent source of vitamins A and C, folate, calcium, and fiber. Look for dark green leaves without yellowing. Collards can be stored in plastic bags in the refrigerator for up to five days.

Manoa lettuce—a mini lettuce with a fresh green hue that's popular in Hawaii where it's grown, manoa lettuce works great in fresh salads and can be substituted for romaine, butter, or any other salad green. Look for fresh leaves without any wilting, and store it, washed and dried, in a plastic bag in the refrigerator for up to five days. Similar to butter lettuce, manoa lettuce is sometimes sold as "living lettuce" with roots still attached to dirt. Store this kind as-is and simply separate and rinse just before using. Manoa lettuce is a vitamin A superstar and also provides vitamin C and folate.

Red leaf lettuce—similar to romaine lettuce, red leaf lettuce is mostly green with red-tipped leaves. It's most commonly enjoyed raw in fresh salads. Red leaf lettuce is rich in vitamins A and K, and a good source of manganese. Rinse and dry leaves on paper towels before storing in plastic bags in the refrigerator for up to a week.

Sorrel—a staple of traditional eastern European and Russian dishes, sorrel is often used as an herb in soups, sauces, and mixed into salads (but it's flavor is too strong to be the base leafy green for a salad). It has a lemony tang that is milder in the spring and more bitter by late fall. Look for green leaves with a fresh scent and avoid brown or wilted leaves. It's best used soon after purchase, but can be stored unwashed in a plastic bag in the refrigerator crisper for up to three days. Sorrel is rich in vitamins A and C, and also provides magnesium and manganese.

Spinach—the workhorse of the leafy greens, spinach deserves its healthy reputation. It's an excellent source of fiber, vitamins A and C, iron, and folate, and provides magnesium. It's been popular in the United States since the early 19th century and is enjoyed both raw in salads or as a cooked side dish. Look for fresh, crisp-looking greens with no evidence of damage from insects. Spinach can be stored in the refrigerator for up to five days, loosely wrapped in damp paper towels and in a plastic bag.

Watercress—a small leafy green that can be mixed into salads and cooked dishes (but not as the main base leafy green), watercress comes from the mustard family and adds a unique bite to any dish. It's an excellent source of vitamins A and C, and a good source of calcium. Watercress should be green without any yellowing or slippery stems, and can be stored up to five days in the refrigerator in a plastic bag after stems are cut, rinsed, and blotted with a paper towel.

Summer Greens

Butter lettuce—see Spring.

Endive—closely related to dandelion, it too has a bite and strong enough flavor to stand up to bold vinaigrettes. Endive can be substituted for dandelion or arugula in recipes. It is fiber-rich and provides vitamin C, calcium, iron, phosphorus, and potassium. Look for crisp and bright green leaves and avoid wilted or browning leaves. It can be stored for up to a week in the refrigerator.

Manoa lettuce—see Spring.

Ong choy spinach—a tropics- and subtropics-loving green, ong choy is also called river spinach or water spinach because it is grown in water. It's popular in Southeast Asian dishes and is commonly used in stir-fry dishes. It looks like a smaller, flatter-leaf spinach, and is an excellent source of iron, vitamins A and C, and a good source of calcium. Look for moist green leaves and stay away from dark, dry, or bruised leaves. Stems should be crisp and green. It's commonly found in Asian markets. Ong choy spinach can be wrapped with damp paper towels and stored in an airtight container in the refrigerator for one to two days.

ARE HERBS AND MICROGREENS HEALTHY?

Herbs and microgreens offer big flavor in a small package. A good rule of thumb is that if a natural food is packing intense color or flavor (or both), it's likely also packing antioxidants and anti-inflammatory compounds.

Many herbs even look like tiny leafy greens, including cilantro, mint, basil, rosemary, sage, oregano, and thyme. Another herb to consider is the perilla leaf, which is about the size of a medium palm, that's related to basil and mint, but uniquely its own flavor. Roll a few perilla leaves into a log and cut them crosswise into thin strips to add to dishes. I like them in salads. Microgreens are in fact tiny, young, leafy greens and often provide multiple times the nutrients of their grown-up counterparts for the same portion size. They offer more intense aromatics, so you can use them like herbs. You may see micro-broccoli, micro-arugula, micro-salad greens mix, and more. Given their small serving size, the nutritional comparison may all even out with the larger greens in a salad. The best way to think of herbs and microgreens is as a way to add interesting textures, flavors, and nutrients to your meals.

Year-Round Vegetables—Beyond Leafy Greens

Bell peppers—whether red, yellow, or green, bell peppers should be heavy for their size with brightly colored tight skin. They can be stored in a plastic bag in the refrigerator for up to five days. Low in calories and high in water and vitamin C, bell peppers are perfect for crudités or stir fries.

Broccoflower—as one would imagine, this is a cross between broccoli and cauliflower, and looks a bit like green cauliflower. Heads should be firm and compact without any brown spots or wilted leaves. It's rich in vitamin C, and provides folate and fiber too. Store refrigerated for up to five days. Enjoy raw, braised, roasted, or sautéed.

Broccolini—sweeter than broccoli due to the cross-breeding with gai lan (see Year-Round Leafy Greens), broccolini stalks are soft and edible. Rich in vitamins A and C, broccolini can be refrigerated in a plastic bag, unwashed, for a week and a half. Its delicate, sweet flavor does well simply steamed or with a quick sauté.

Carrots—these can be orange, purple, white, red, or yellow. Look for smooth, firm, crisp carrots with deep color and fresh green tops. Avoid soft, wilted, or split carrots. They're rich in vitamins A and C.

Celeriac—also known as celery root, celeriac is rough and knobby with an uneven surface and mottled brown-white outer layer. Peel the outer layer away to expose a creamy white interior that can be chopped up and used like potatoes—in home fries, roasted, or pureed into soups. It can also be made into a mash, or the raw form can be sliced thin for slaws and salads. Store in the refrigerator for up to a week. It's rich in vitamins C and K, and a good source of fiber and potassium.

Celery—an underrated vegetable, celery offers a satisfying, crisp crunch along with vitamins A and C. Look for straight, rigid stalks with fresh leaves. Refrigerate for up to a week or more. Try celery stalks with French mustard for a simple snack.

Cherry tomatoes—store at room temperature away from direct sunlight and enjoy within a week after ripening; they taste best unrefrigerated. Rich in vitamins A and C, cherry tomatoes also provide vitamin K and potassium. Versatile, they can be tossed into pasta sauces, soups, and salads, or enjoyed raw for a snack.

Chinese eggplant—purple and the shape of a small zucchini, Chinese eggplant is sweeter and more tender than conventional eggplant and can be cooked without peeling or salting, so you get the benefit of the polyphenols in the skin. Look for eggplant that is heavy for its size with firm, glossy skin. Refrigerate and use within a week.

Leeks—related to onions, leeks have a nuanced, sweeter flavor. They look like large green onions with white bulbs and green tops. Leeks are rich in vitamin A and a good source of folate and vitamin C. Store them unwashed in a plastic bag for up to two weeks. Thinly slice the white bulb to add to savory dishes, and slice the green tops for garnish.

Mushrooms—rich in a satisfying umami flavor, mushrooms make a nutritious and flavorful meat alternative. They're low in calories, a good source of B vitamins, and contain some vitamin D. Look for mushrooms that are firm, without spots or slime.

Onions—offering immense flavor without the salt, onions are an unsung hero of delicious dishes. They're also high in vitamin C and a good source of fiber. Onions should be stored similar to potatoes, in a cool, dark, well-ventilated place for up to four weeks. Cut onions can be stored in the refrigerator for use within two to three days.

Parsnips—pale white and shaped like large carrots, parsnips should be firm and dry without pits. Look for smaller ones for a flavorful and more tender treat. A good source of vitamin C, folate, and fiber, parsnips' sugar develops with cold weather, so though they are available year-round, try them in the late fall, after a frost. Store in the produce drawer for two to three weeks.

Pearl onions—about the size of a large marble and commonly eaten whole, pearl onions are otherwise like regular onions and come in white, yellow, and red varieties, and pack flavor and vitamin C. Look for onions that are dry with papery skins still attached.

Potatoes—high in vitamin C and potassium. Look for potatoes that are clean, firm, smooth, dry, and uniform in size. They can be stored in a cool, dry, well-ventilated place for three to five weeks.

Starchy russets are best for mashing, and waxy Yukon Gold, red, white, and fingerling potatoes are better for roasting. Purple potatoes are great for steaming or baking.

Snow peas—shiny and flat, with small peas in the pod, snow peas should be stored unwashed in a perforated bag in the refrigerator for up to a week. They are mild and slightly sweet, and can be enjoyed raw, steamed, stir fried, or mixed into salads or pasta dishes.

Yucca root—brown on the outside, white on the inside, vitamin C-rich yucca root can be used in soups in place of potatoes. Store in a cool, dark, dry place for up to a week, or peel, wrap tightly, and store in the freezer for several months.

Fall Vegetables

Acorn squash—shaped like an acorn, it even has a mildly nutty flavor. The skin should be dull, without any soft spots or cracks. As with other squash, look for something heavy for its size. Store away from extreme temperatures and sunlight, in a cool, dry area. It can stay fresh for up to three months. It's a good source of vitamin C and only 30 calories per half cup.

Black salsify—also known as an oyster plant because of the root's oyster-like flavor. Meanwhile, the leaves, if attached, can be used as a salad green. The long root should have a black skin and creamy interior. Look for smooth and firm roots. Cut off the root end, peel off the outer skin, spritz with lemon juice to keep it from browning, cube it and add to soups, or boil and mash like potatoes. Avoid overcooking, as it can become stringy and mushy.

Broccoli—super nutritious, broccoli is rich in vitamin C and folate, and a good source of fiber and potassium. The heads should be tight and florets should be bluish-green. Refrigerate and use within three to five days.

Brussels sprouts—they look like little baby cabbages and are a related vegetable. These little cruciferous vegetables are low in calories and high in vitamin C, folate, fiber, and so much more. Look for firm, compact, bright green brussels sprouts, on the stalk if possible. Simply toss with extra-virgin olive oil, vinegar, salt, and pepper, and roast for a delicious side dish. They last refrigerated for up to a week.

Buttercup squash–a sweet, creamy orange squash, the skin of buttercup squash is dark green. Look for a squash that is heavy for its size with an even color. They can be stored in a cool, dry place for up to three months.

Butternut squash–with flesh that is a vibrant orange like pumpkin, butternut squash can be used in any recipe that calls for pumpkin. Store in a cool, dark place for up to a month. It's an excellent source of vitamins A and C, and a good source of fiber, potassium, and magnesium.

Cardoon–with a flavor that's like a blend of artichokes and celery, cardoon looks like oversized celery. A good source of potassium, magnesium, and folate, cardoon can be enjoyed cooked or raw in salads.

Cauliflower–high in vitamin C and a good source of folate, cauliflower should have compact, white curds and bright green, firmly attached leaves. Avoid brown spots or loose sections. Refrigerate in a plastic bag for up to five days. Enjoy it roasted or experiment with cauliflower "mashed potatoes" or "rice."

Chayote squash–use anywhere summer squash would be a good fit.

Chinese long beans–these can measure up to 3 feet long, with a taste similar to green beans, and can be prepared in similar ways. However, they are more flexible (less crisp). Refrigerate in a plastic bag for up to five days. They're rich in iron, fiber, folate, potassium, and zinc. They're also a source of calcium.

Delicata squash–also known as the peanut squash and Bohemian squash, it is an elongated squash that should appear light yellow with green striations when ripe, and light green when unripe. Rich in vitamin A. Look for squash that is heavy for its size. Delicata squash hold their shape when cooked, making them perfect for stuffing with whole grains, lean poultry, and vegetables.

Daikon radish—long, white, and slender, the daikon radish should be shiny, firm, and smooth. It's low in calories and a good source of vitamin C. Store it tightly wrapped in plastic in the refrigerator for up to three days. With a mild peppery bite, they can be used in any recipe that calls for radishes.

Garlic—so much flavor comes out of these small, white bulbs, and their sulfuric compounds are being studied for a variety of health benefits. Store in a cool, dark place, outside the refrigerator, for several weeks. Try chopping off the top of a whole bulb and roasting with extra-virgin olive oil, wrapped up in foil, until the cloves become soft, mild in flavor, and spreadable.

Ginger—a flavorful root, ginger is simply amazing and adds depth of flavor and aromatics to any dish. Look for firm roots with smooth skin and a spicy aroma. Avoid cracked or withered ginger. A good source of vitamin C, magnesium, potassium, and plenty of polyphenols, ginger can be peeled and chopped, then added to stir-fry dishes, pasta sauces, smoothies, and even turkey patties.

Hearts of Palm—harvested from the central core of palm trees, they are soft and firm at the same time and offer a mildly sweet taste. They are available fresh, but are more commonly found canned or jarred, and work well sliced into salads or pureed into soups and sauces. If fresh, refrigerate immediately in a tightly sealed container for up to two weeks. Packaged hearts of palm should be stored away from direct sunlight and will stay fresh for about a week after opening. Hearts of palm are rich in potassium, vitamin C, iron, copper, zinc, and B vitamins.

Jerusalem artichoke—looking nothing like an artichoke and related to sunflowers, which is why they are also known as sunchokes, Jerusalem artichokes are starchy tubers like potatoes or turnips. Look for firm, relatively smooth skin, and store in a plastic bag in the refrigerator for up to a week. They're a good source of iron. When roasted, the skin gets flaky and the flesh tender. The taste is slightly nutty and sweet.

Pumpkin—Indigenous to North America, pumpkins aren't just for Halloween decor. They're an excellent source of vitamin A and a good source of vitamin C. Look for pumpkins that are heavy for their size, and store in a cool, dark place for up to two months. Roast, cube, and add to salads, or roast, puree, and add to smoothies, muffins, and breads.

Sweet potatoes—A truly misunderstood vegetable, they're not actually related to potatoes and sometimes mislabeled as yams. High in vitamins A and C and a good source of potassium, sweet potatoes should be stored in a cool, dark place for up to three to five weeks. Bake, roast, or steam them, and use them in salads, puree them into pancakes, or enjoy them on their own.

Turnips—Though they come in all shapes and colors, you're most likely to see the purple and white variety. Look for heavy turnips, and keep in mind that the smaller ones are sweeter. They can be eaten raw or cooked and are rich in vitamin C. They can be stored in the refrigerator for a few days, but they get bitter with longer storage.

Winter Vegetables

Brussels sprouts—see Fall.
   Buttercup squash—see Fall.
   Cardoon—see Fall.
   Delicata squash—see Fall.
   Sweet potatoes—see Fall.
   Turnips—see Fall.

Spring Vegetables

Artichokes—choose plump, tight artichokes that are heavy for their size. They're a good source of vitamin C, fiber, folate, and magnesium.

Store them refrigerated for up to a week and keep dry. Don't toss the stem; that's where the tender and delicious heart extends.

Asparagus—available in green, purple, and white, but the green variety is often the most tender. The slimmer the stalk, the more delicate the flavor. Look for firm stalks with tight tips, and stay away from any that are limp or wilted. Wrap the ends of the stalks in a wet paper towel, and store in a plastic bag, refrigerated, for up to four days. Diagonally sliced, one-inch pieces of asparagus, lightly sautéed, are a gorgeous and healthy add-in to warm grain salads.

Chayote squash—see Fall.

Fennel—sometimes called sweet anise, fennel has a delicate licorice aroma and flavor. Their feathery tops can be used like an herb, and the firm white bulbs can be sliced into salads, made into slaw, sautéed, or roasted with extra-virgin olive oil. Keep it refrigerated and use within five days. Fennel is a good source of vitamin C, potassium, and fiber.

Fiddlehead ferns—so named as they resemble the curved decorative end of a fiddle, the season for this spring green is short, but worth staying vigilant for. Look for a tight coil with only an inch or two uncoiled, bright color, and firmness. Best to enjoy them as soon as possible, but they should last in the refrigerator, wrapped to avoid drying out, for up to three days. They can be prepared similarly to asparagus. Simple methods are best so that their seasonal flavor can shine through.

Green beans—also known as string beans, green beans can be eaten fresh or cooked. Look for green beans with good color that are firm enough that they would snap easily when bent. Refrigerate and use within a week. They're a good source of vitamin C and fiber.

Morel mushrooms—a springtime darling, morel mushroom caps look like honeycombs. They should smell fresh and earthy, without soft spots, bruising, or slime. Store them, unwashed, in a paper bag in the refrigerator for up to three days. They're an excellent source of vitamin D.

Peas—also known as sweet peas or English peas, they can be enjoyed raw or cooked. They should be firm, bright green, and medium in size. They can be refrigerated in a perforated plastic bag for three to five days. Shell just before using. Peas are a good source of vitamin A, folate, and fiber.

Vidalia onions—Georgia's official state vegetable, the Vidalia onion is sweet and savory all at the same time. They're sweet due to lower sulfur in the Georgia soil they're grown in. They can be enjoyed raw in salads, roasted, grilled, or caramelized. Like other onions, they're a good source of vitamin C.

Summer Vegetables

Armenian cucumber—about 12 to 15 inches long and pale green, this cuke is actually a melon with a mild cucumber taste. It requires no deseeding or peeling, and can be used raw in drinks, appetizers, salads, snacks, or cooked like zucchini. A good source of water and vitamin C, store them in the refrigerator crisper for a few days.

Beets—they can't be beat. Look for firm, smooth-skinned beets, and know that the smaller they are in size, the more tender they'll be. An excellent source of folate and polyphenols, beets have an earthy, sweet flavor. They can be boiled or roasted, and the greens can be enjoyed raw or sautéed. Store in a plastic bag, refrigerated, for up to three weeks.

Chinese long beans—see Fall.

Corn—there's nothing like fresh, sweet summer corn. Look for green husks, fresh silks, and tight rows of kernels. Refrigerate with husks on and use as soon as possible, within one to two days. An easy way to prepare corn is to steam or boil it until it simply smells like corn. Corn is a good source of vitamin C.

Crookneck squash—a vitamin C-rich yellow summer squash that is quick cooking, crookneck squash is best when no bigger than 8 inches around. Like other squashes, choose one that is heavy for its size. Refrigerate for up to a week.

Cucumbers—crisp and mildly sweet, cucumbers should be firm, evenly shaped, and dark green in color. Look for cucumbers that are heavy for their size, and store them refrigerated, bagged, for up to a week. Cucumbers are a good source of vitamin C, are water-packed, and have natural cooling agents. Enjoy them raw as a simple snack, in salads, in cucumber sandwiches, or scoop out the seeds to make cucumber cups and fill with hummus for an easy appetizer.

Eggplant—look for eggplants that are heavy for their size, without discoloration. They can be stored in the crisper for five to seven days. Due to their meaty and toothsome texture, eggplants are a popular center-of-plate item for plant-based eaters. They soak up flavor like a sponge.

French beans—similar to but slimmer than green beans, they are also known as haricots verts. French beans should be bright in color and crisp. Store them in a plastic bag, refrigerated, for one to two weeks. They're an excellent source of fiber, B vitamins, folate, magnesium, and potassium. Try them blanched and added to salads, alongside Ahi tuna steaks, or in an Asian stir-fry dish.

Garlic—see Fall.

Grape tomatoes—see Year-Round Vegetables, Cherry tomatoes.

Green beans—see Spring.

Hearts of Palm—see Fall.

Okra—slippery when cooked, okra tastes great paired with tomatoes in stews. Look for firm, brightly colored pods and refrigerate for up to three days. Okra is an excellent source of vitamin C, and a good source of folate and fiber.

Peas—see Spring.

Radishes—rich in vitamin C, radishes are crisp and peppery, adding a bright note to any salad or savory dish. Tops should be green and fresh, roots should be smooth and bright. They can be refrigerated in a plastic bag for use within a week.

Shallots—related to onions, but more delicate, sweet, and mild, shallots should be firm and heavy for their size, with dry, papery skins. They can be stored in a cool, dark, well-ventilated place for up to four weeks. Cut shallots should be refrigerated, tightly sealed, and used within two to three days. They are a good source of vitamins A and C.

Sugar snap peas—enjoy as soon as possible to get a sweet, crisp taste, which diminishes with storage time. They can be kept in the crisper in a perforated plastic bag for up to two days. Sugar snap peas are rich in vitamin C and a good source of vitamin K. Simply pull back the fibrous seam and enjoy them as a fresh snack.

Tomatillo—also known as tomate verde and Mexican husk tomato, the tomatillo is a small, green tomato surrounded by a papery husk. Look for dry, hard tomatillos with tight husks. They can be refrigerated in the crisper for two to three weeks. An excellent source of vitamin C, one of the easiest and tastiest ways to enjoy them is in salsas. Simply peel away the papery skin, and puree with onions, peppers, cilantro, and a pinch of salt.

Tomatoes—look for bright, shiny skins and firm flesh, and store away from direct sunlight. They should be enjoyed within a week after ripening and taste best when not refrigerated. They are rich in vitamins A and C, and provide lycopene and potassium.

Yukon Gold potatoes—a cross between the North American white potato and a wild South American yellow potato, Yukons are rich in vitamin C and a good source of potassium. Store them in a cool, dark, well-ventilated place and use within three to five weeks. They are waxy with a firm texture, making them great for roasting, soups, stews, and gratins because they keep their shape.

Zucchini—a summer squash, zucchini skin should be firm, slightly prickly, shiny, and free from cuts or bruises. Zucchini can be stored in the refrigerator, in a plastic bag, for four to five days. It is high in vitamin C and quick cooking, making it ideal for a stir fry, chopped into an omelet, added to casseroles and sauces, or simply grilled.

Whole Grains

Whole grains are an important part of the daily diet in the MIND, Mediterranean, and DASH diets. Whole grains are a kind of seed. To be considered whole, a grain must contain all of the essential parts and naturally occurring nutrition of the entire seed or kernel, including all of the germ seed, fleshy endosperm, and outer bran. Whole grains provide an excellent source of vitamin E, which has been proven to protect the brain.

Evidence suggests whole grains have always played a key role in brain health, starting as early as millions of years ago. Researchers in Europe and Australia studied the role of diet with early humans, noting that carbs from whole grains, roots, and starchy plant foods were required to support the increased metabolic demands of a growing brain. While many people associate early humans with meat-based diets, it was actually cooked starches that helped accelerate brain size starting in the Middle Pleistocene time.

Today, whole grains are being studied for benefits for cardiovascular disease, diabetes, cancers, cognitive health, and more. According to the Whole Grains Council, "because of the phytochemicals and antioxidants, people who eat three daily servings of whole grains have been shown to reduce their risk of heart disease by 25 to 36 percent, stroke by 37 percent, type 2 diabetes by 21 to 27 percent, digestive system cancers by 21 to 43 percent, and hormone-related cancers by 10 to 40 percent."

Cognitive benefits of eating whole grains may start early. In a 2015 study, elementary school students scored higher in all areas of testing after eating breakfast. Those who ate more whole grains had significantly higher scores in reading comprehension, verbal fluency, and math. Whole grains also play a role in neuroprotection later in life.

One study of more than 2,000 older Swedish adults suggests that neuroprotective diets should include whole grains, vegetables, nuts, legumes, and fish, while unhealthy diets included foods such as refined grains, processed foods, red meat, and sugar. Another study found that the anti-inflammatory protection provided by whole grains slowed cognitive decline among more than 5,000 middle-aged adults. Not surprisingly, the highest levels of inflammation were linked to diets high in red meat and fried food, and lower in whole grains. The bottom line is that overall diet patterns higher in whole grains are shown to slow cognitive decline.

Cooking grains is a simple proposition, and the main downside is the time it takes. A little preplanning can take care of this. However, for the days when you need whole grains in a hurry, there are high-quality frozen and 10-minute par-cooked whole grains on the market with little to no nutritional compromise. From ancient grains to modern quick-cooking versions, whole grains have a lot to offer.

Amaranth—a small, gluten-free, ancient pseudo-grain, amaranth is higher in protein than most other grains at 14 percent, and contains lysine, an amino acid not commonly found in grains. It has a nutty, peppery flavor and a crunchy texture at its center, even when fully cooked, making it ideal for adding to salads and baked goods. Amaranth is most often if not always sold in whole grain form. Prepare 6 cups of water to 1 cup of dry amaranth, then drain. A Half cup, cooked serving is a good source of iron and magnesium.

Barley—a fiber superstar, barley is 17 to 30 percent fiber (by comparison, whole wheat is 12 percent fiber, oats are 10 percent fiber, and corn is 7 percent fiber). Generally, a grain's fiber is in its outer bran layer. Interestingly, in barley, fiber is found throughout the grain, so even refined barley will have some fiber. Still, look for whole grain barley labeled with terms such as "whole barley," "dehulled barley," "hulled barley," or "hull-less barley," and bypass the refined versions that may be labeled as "pearled" or "quick-cooking" barley.

Buckwheat—previously known as a poor man's food, it grows well on rocky hillsides and is hardy enough to thrive without pesticides. Today it enjoys health food chic and has gotten attention for containing the antioxidant rutin, which may improve circulation. Like amaranth, buckwheat is not a true grain and is not even wheat, despite its name. In fact, unlike all true wheat varieties, buckwheat is gluten-free. Japanese soba noodles are traditionally made with buckwheat; it is also used in crepes.

Bulgur—when wheat kernels have been boiled, dried, and cracked, the result is bulgur. Because it has already been precooked and dried, prepare it like dry pasta because it's ready after about 10 minutes of boiling. It's commonly used in a dish called tabbouleh, a grain salad with bulgur, mint, parsley, tomatoes, extra-virgin olive oil, and lemon juice. Bulgur provides more fiber than quinoa, oats, millet, buckwheat, or corn.

Corn—more commonly thought of as a movie theater snack or summer picnic vegetable, corn is still in fact a whole grain. DNA testing shows corn originally came from Mexico, where it was developed into an agricultural staple about 9,000 years ago. Corn is a gluten-free grain that provides more vitamin A and related carotenoids than most other grains.

It gets a bad rap as most of the corn in the US and Canada is used to feed animals (called dent or field corn), but there are other unique varieties that have a role in human diets. Sweet corn is the kind that is in season in the summer and can be eaten off the cob. It should be eaten soon after harvesting because the sugars start converting to starches as soon as it's picked. If you need to store it, leave it in the husk.

When eaten with beans, corn helps provide complete proteins. In traditional Central and South American culinary cultures, corn is commonly soaked in lime water, which adds calcium and increases B-vitamin absorption. Corn products that commonly go through this process are masa flour, tortillas, and the southern US's hominy.

Einkorn—an ancient wheat variety that fell out of favor as a mainstream crop because of how difficult it is to remove its hull, einkorn is still grown in some areas of Europe, and more recently has had a resurgence in Washington state. Einkorn is a drought-tolerant grain that is just about always in whole grain form. Among wheat varieties, it has the highest levels of carotenoids such as lutein, zeaxanthin, and beta-carotene. Though it still contains gluten and the wheat protein gliadin, einkorn is less allergenic compared to other types of wheat.

Farro (aka Emmer)—farro, as it's known in Italy, is another ancient wheat variety and was one of the first domesticated grains grown in the Fertile Crescent in the Middle East (modern-day Iraq, Syria, Lebanon, Jordan, Israel, and Egypt). It has higher total antioxidant activity than other wheats. Similar to einkorn, farro is harder to hull than modern durum wheat, which is why it fell out of favor. Farro comes pearled (i.e., refined) and in whole-grain forms, so be sure to choose whole grain farro. There are quick-cooking whole grain farro options on the market.

Freekeh—yet another kind of wheat, freekeh is also known as farik and frikeh, and is often sold cracked into smaller quick-cooking pieces the way bulgur wheat is. Freekeh is usually made from hard durum wheat, harvested when still young and green, then roasted and rubbed. Freekeh has a smoky flavor, and works well in Middle Eastern and North African cuisine, including pilafs, grain salads, and porridges. It is commonly sold in whole grain form.

Fonio—Fonio is an ancient whole grain native to West Africa, with small grains that cook in five minutes. It is considered the oldest cultivated grain in Africa. Other names for fonio are acha, iburura, and hungry rice. It's drought tolerant and also naturally gluten-free. Fonio is a good source of B-vitamins and calcium. It can be used in pilafs, porridges, and in many dishes as an alternative to rice or couscous.

Khorasan wheat—an ancient wheat variety whose name comes from the ancient Egyptian name for wheat, and is about two to three times the size of most wheats. It that has enjoyed a recent return to the US food supply. It has a nutty taste and is higher in protein than other wheat because it has never been hybridized. Look for whole Kamut to make sure you're getting whole grains. It can be found whole or as flour in natural food stores, and is also in some commercial products such as pasta, puffed cereal, and crackers.

Kaniwa (cousins with quinoa)—like quinoa, kaniwa (alternatively spelled qaniwa, canihua, and canahua) is a tiny pseudo-grain that is high in protein. It comes from the cold mountains of Peru and Bolivia. Unlike quinoa, kaniwa doesn't need to be rinsed as thoroughly, as it's not coated with the bitter substances that need to be washed off of quinoa (called saponins). It is labor-intensive to harvest and is traditionally lightly roasted and ground into a flour before being consumed in hot and cold drinks and porridges. Since it's a specialty item, it will most likely be sold in whole grain form, whether the word "whole" is used on the label or not. Kaniwa is gluten-free.

Millet—millet isn't just one grain. Millet includes a group of related grains from around the world. Other names for millet are pearl millet, foxtail millet, proso millet (also called hog, common, or broom corn millet), finger millet (also called ragi), and fonio. Millet is common in India, China, South America, Russia, and the Himalayas. Millet comes in white, gray, yellow, or red varieties, and is just about always in whole grain form. India is the world's largest millet producer, where it is used to make roti, a common flatbread. It can also be used in pilafs, breakfast porridges, added to breads and soups, or popped like popcorn. It's gluten-free and high in magnesium and antioxidants.

Oats—oats need no introduction, as just about everyone in the United States has encountered oatmeal for breakfast at one time or another. Though oats are processed in a variety of ways, their bran and germ aren't typically removed, so just about all oats on the market are in whole grain form. Most are steamed and flattened into soft, quick-cooking oats, also known as "old-fashioned," "regular," or "rolled" oats. These are the kind of oats found in instant oatmeal. For a nuttier flavor and more toothsome texture, try steel cut oats, which are sometimes called Irish or Scottish oats. To get to steel cut oats, the entire oat (which looks like a grain of rice) is sliced a couple times into smaller pieces for quicker (but not instant) cooking that takes about 20 minutes. Steel cut oatmeal is an entirely different experience compared to rolled oats.

Oats contain a soluble fiber called beta-glucan that helps lower cholesterol. They also contain antioxidants that may help protect blood vessels from LDL cholesterol damage. They can be enjoyed as the traditional breakfast porridge, in a pilaf dinner side dish, mixed into turkey burgers, or as a crispy coating for baked chicken.

Quinoa—an ancient Incan pseudo-grain from the Andes mountains, quinoa provides a complete protein and cooks in about 10 to 12 minutes, making it a convenient and super-nutritious vegetarian protein choice. It keeps its texture well, so it works great in pilafs, soups, and salads. It is a very small, round grain that has a little "tail" that pops out when it's finished cooking. Most quinoa must be rinsed before cooking to wash away bitter residue from compounds called saponins. Quinoa comes in many colors, including red, purple, orange, green, black, and yellow.

Rice—whole grain rice is usually brown but can also be black, purple, or red, and comes in long-, medium-, or short-grain forms. The top rice-growing states in the United States are Arkansas, California, Louisiana, Mississippi, Missouri, and Texas, where rice-friendly warm, humid climates are available. Rice cookers are extremely convenient. Simply measure out the rice and water, press cook, and you're done. Make a large batch of whole grain rice and enjoy over a couple days. Rice is naturally gluten-free.

Rye—related to wheat and long considered to be a weed, it became valued for its ability to grow quickly and in climates too wet, cold, or drought-affected for other grains. It is a traditional staple in northern Europe, Russia, Poland, Canada, Argentina, China, and Turkey. Look for whole rye or rye berries to ensure it is a whole grain. Rye contains a high level of fiber in both its bran and its inner endosperm, and is most commonly enjoyed as bread or crisp bread, but can also be used in soups and grain salads.

Sorghum—also known as milo, guinea corn, kaffir corn, durra, mtama, jowar, and kaoliang—sorghum is an ancient grain that grows well in the Great Plains, from South Dakota to Texas. Nearly always sold in its whole grain form whether it's labeled "whole" or not, sorghum is gluten-free and grown from traditional seeds, so it's naturally non-GMO. Most of the sorghum in the United States goes to animal feed or made into biodegradable packing materials. However, it can be eaten as a porridge or popped like popcorn.

Spelt—a higher-protein variety of wheat, spelt can replace wheat in most recipes. In Italy it is known as farro grande (that is, big farro). Spelt is sold in both whole and refined form, so be sure to look for whole spelt.

Teff—a tiny-sized grain that is common in Ethiopia, it is used to make the spongy, pleasantly sour flatbread called injera. Teff is a kind of millet and grows in red, purple, gray, yellowy brown, and ivory colors. It grows well in both flood and drought conditions, from sea level to mile-high altitudes. Teff is higher in calcium and resistant starch (a type of dietary fiber) than other grains. In fact, a cup of cooked teff has about the same amount of calcium as a half cup of cooked spinach. It can be enjoyed in porridges, polenta, crepes, and breads. It cooks quickly, offers a mild flavor, and is gluten-free. It is almost always sold in whole grain form.

Triticale—compared to all the ancient grains available, the wheat-rye hybrid triticale is a baby. Commercially grown triticale has only been around for a few decades. Rye and wheat easily cross-breed in nature, and the resulting triticale grows well without industrial fertilizers and pesticides, which makes it a good option for organic farmers. As a blend of both rye and wheat, triticale contains gluten.

Wheat—while gluten is harmful to people who are allergic to it, gluten is also the reason wheat became so valuable to bread bakers since it helps them create toothsome risen breads. There are two main varieties of wheat—hard winter durum wheat (used commonly for pasta) and soft spring bread wheat (used most often for most other wheat foods). Hard wheat has more protein and more gluten than spring wheat, making it ideal for bread baking. Soft wheat creates cake flour. It also comes in red and white varieties that refer to their color, not whether they're whole grain or not, which means it's possible to have whole white wheat made from whole grain soft white wheat. To be sure you're getting a whole grain, look for the word "whole" on the label. Wheat varieties and hybrids include wheat berries, bulgur, farro, einkorn, spelt, Kamut, durum, red wheat, white wheat, spring wheat, winter wheat, and triticale.

Wild rice—not technically rice, it is native to the Americas and was originally grown around the Great Lakes. Today, most wild rice is still harvested by Native Americans in the Minnesota area, though it's also grown and harvested to a lesser extent in California and elsewhere in the Midwest. Wild rice has a pleasantly strong nutty flavor and firm texture, with twice the protein and fiber of brown rice (but less iron and calcium). Wild rice is just about always sold as a whole grain, and is a good source of fiber, folate, magnesium, zinc, vitamin B6, and niacin. It works great in stuffed mushrooms, grain salads, and soups, and can be popped like popcorn.

What are Sprouted Whole Grains?

Grains used to sprout accidentally, but most grains today no longer do so by happenstance. There may be some nutritional benefits to sprouting a grain, which has led some food producers and home experimenters to purposefully sprout their grains.

The germ of a whole grain is the plant embryo, and it feeds on the starchy endosperm and bran of a whole grain until it's ready to germinate into a new plant. When temperature and moisture conditions are just right, the whole grain will sprout. When sprouting starts, enzymes make the endosperm starch easier for the germ to digest; some people may also find this "activated" type of grain easier to digest as well.

When a grain is properly and safely sprouted, it's both seed and new plant, which makes it more digestible and higher in vitamins and minerals such as B vitamins, vitamin C, folate, fiber, and an amino acid often lacking in grains, lysine.

Keep in mind that the process requires precision in the time, temperature, and moisture used. Too much moisture and the grain drowns and opens from swelling versus sprouting, and can ferment or even rot. Left for too long, a healthy sprout can continue to grow into a new grass stalk, which is not very digestible to humans.

If interested in sprouted grains, look for a brand you trust to sprout their grains under carefully controlled conditions. Remember, sprouted or not, whole grains are an extremely healthy food choice.

Nuts

The MIND diet recommends eating nuts most days (at least five times a week), in part because nuts are a rich source of vitamin E, a nutrient that protects the brain. In addition, walnuts are unique among nuts for offering an excellent source of omega-3 fatty acids. Nuts also have a clear and well-established role in heart health. In 2003, the FDA approved the following claim: "Scientific evidence suggests but does not prove that eating 1½ ounces per day of most nuts as part of a diet low in saturated fat and cholesterol may reduce the risk of heart disease." Previous and ongoing research shows that nuts are protective for diabetes, cancers, longevity, and cognitive health.

A 2013 randomized clinical trial in Spain, called PREDIMED-NAVARRA, showed that following a Mediterranean diet with either extra nuts or olive oil resulted in higher cognitive scores compared to low-fat diets. The study participants included 522 men and women at high risk for cardiovascular disease who were on average 75 years of age. After six and a half years of being on either a Mediterranean diet with additional olive oil, or a Mediterranean diet with additional nuts, participants had significantly higher global cognitive scores compared to the low-fat control diet.

How do nuts slow down cognitive decline? To find out, the USDA reviewed several studies focusing on almonds, pecans, pistachios, and walnuts, and found that these tree nuts slow down age-related cognitive decline, perhaps because they reduce oxidative stress and inflammation. Nuts are nutrient-dense and contain a variety of bioactive compounds, including polyunsaturated fats, phytochemicals, and polyphenols. In addition to vitamin E, they provide folate, fiber, and flavonoids, such as proanthocyanidins.

In addition to cognitive health, nuts have a role in overall health and longevity. Harvard researchers examining decades of data from more than 76,000 women and more than 42,000 men in the United States found that the more nuts people ate, the longer they lived. Compared to people who didn't eat nuts, people who ate nuts seven or more times per week had a 20 percent lower death rate from heart disease, cancer, and respiratory diseases. These findings are supported by earlier studies finding longevity benefits for whites, blacks, and elderly people at five servings of nuts per week, and at three servings per week for Spanish adults at risk for heart disease.

Should you be worried about nuts and weight gain? The short answer is no. Eating nuts more often is associated with less weight gain, reduced belly fat, and a lower risk for obesity. That being said, food choices should always fit within appropriate calorie ranges.

Eating nuts at least five times a week works out nicely for a daily work-week snack habit. Nuts are antioxidant-rich nuggets of good health, and very versatile in the kitchen. They can be added to vegetable dishes, morning oatmeal, chopped and used to crust fish, in salads and stir-fry dishes, in salad dressings, or simply on their own as a healthy snack.

When selecting in-shell nuts, they should feel heavy for their size. Avoid nuts with signs of insect or moisture damage, or that rattle when shaken, which is a sign they have dried out and are old. Shells should not have holes, and should not have cracks, except pistachios, which naturally open part way.

For packages of shelled nuts (kernels), look for expiration dates, avoid nuts that look rubbery or shriveled, and smell them to make sure they're not rancid. Store nuts in an airtight container in a cool dry place. They can also be refrigerated or frozen.

All nuts provide healthy unsaturated fats, and for the most part there is a good ratio of more unsaturated to less saturated fat. Some nuts contain more saturated fat than others. The easiest way to ensure you're not going overboard on saturated fat is to simply mix it up and eat a variety of nuts.

The following nuts contain a higher percentage of healthy unsaturated fats, and less than 2 grams of saturated fat per 1-ounce serving: almonds, hazelnuts, pine nuts, pistachios, and walnuts.

Health Nuts

Almonds—eighty percent of the world's almond supply is grown in California's Central Valley, and at 23 almonds per serving, whole almonds are a satisfying snack. They are known for being rich in vitamin E and a good source of calcium. They're also a good source of folate, magnesium, and fiber. They last up to a year in the refrigerator.

Hazelnuts—also known as filberts, a serving is 21 nuts. The hazelnut grows in temperate climates and is the official state nut of Oregon, which grows 95 percent of the US commercial crop. They're rich in vitamin E, copper, and manganese, and a good source of magnesium and fiber. They can be stored up to three months out of the refrigerator, up to six months in the refrigerator, and up to a year frozen. Hazelnuts pair with savory, citrus, and sweet flavors.

Pine nuts—also known as Indian nut, piñon, pinoli, and pignolia, pine nuts are the soft nuts found inside of pine cones. They are widely used in Mediterranean dishes and commonly used in the United States as a garnish or blended into pestos. Pine nuts are a good source of vitamin E and number 167 nuts per ounce.

Pistachios—California is one of the world's top pistachio producers and grows 98 percent of the US crop. Pistachios are green due to chlorophyll, lutein, and zeaxanthin. They're a good source of protein, fiber, magnesium, manganese, copper, thiamin, and phosphorus. There are 49 nuts in a serving.

Walnuts—the only nut with a significant amount of omega-3 fats, walnuts are rich in manganese and copper, and a good source of magnesium. The fertile land in California's Central Valley grows 99 percent of the US supply and three-quarters of global trade. They can be stored in the refrigerator for up to three months and up to a year in the freezer. There are 14 halves per serving.

Other Nuts

Brazil nuts—there are six nuts per serving, as Brazils are large. As one might imagine from their name, these nuts grow in the Amazon. About 15 to 25 nuts grow inside a shell about the size of a coconut. They last out of the refrigerator in a cool, dry place for up to a month, or frozen for up to a year. Brazils are known for providing a full day's worth of selenium, an antioxidant. They're also rich in magnesium, copper, and phosphorus, and a good source of manganese, vitamin E, and thiamin.

Cashews—a single cashew nut dangles from an apple-shaped fruit before it is harvested. Soft with a delicate flavor, cashews are native to South America. Today, most are grown in India, Brazil, Vietnam, and Mozambique. They can be used to create creamy nut butters and vegan cheese. Cashews are rich in copper and a good source of magnesium, manganese, vitamin K, phosphorus, and zinc. They last in the refrigerator for up to six months, and up to a year frozen. There are 18 nuts per serving.

Macadamia nuts—There are 10 to 12 nuts per serving of these smooth buttery nuts that grow natively in Australia and Hawaii. They're an excellent source of manganese and a good source of thiamin. They should be refrigerated and can last up to two months there, or in unopened, airtight containers for up to a year in the freezer.

Pecans—with 19 halves per serving, pecans are native to what is now the United States South. They are commonly used in sweets, but a healthier way to enjoy them is as a simple snack, a fish crust, or in a green salad. Pecans are rich in manganese, and a good source of copper, thiamin, and fiber. They last for up to six months refrigerated, and up to a year frozen.

Peanuts—not technically a nut (they're a legume), they have many of the same properties and health benefits as tree nuts. They go by other names, like groundnut and goober. They're an excellent source of manganese and a good source of folate, magnesium, phosphorus, vitamin E, and niacin. There are 28 kernels per serving.

Seeds

Though not technically nuts, seeds offer many of the same nutrients as nuts, which is why you'll often see "nuts and seeds" discussed together. They're concentrated sources of essential nutrients. Here are a few examples.

Chia seeds—A tiny seed thought to be native to Central America, chia seeds are often available in black or white varieties. A tablespoon is about half an ounce, which is a good source of fiber and anti-inflammatory omega-3s. A little more than half of its healthy fats come from omega-3 ALA. They absorb water to form a gel in minutes, so they work well to add bulk to overnight oats, smoothies, and chia puddings. They can be soaked overnight in the refrigerator.

Flaxseed—Small shiny dark brown seeds with an almond shape, flaxseed are a source of plant-based omega-3s, which soothe inflammation and are tied to better brain health as well as heart health. A one tablespoon serving is also a good source of the B-vitamin thiamine, which is essential to cognitive health. Flaxseed must be ground before its nutrients are available. Otherwise, their hard exteriors mean they pass through the digestive system largely intact. Flaxseed is sold ground or can be ground at home in a spice or coffee grinder. Grounds should be stored in the refrigerator to keep them fresher for longer, and if grinding at home, only do a small amount at a time since it accelerates its perishability.

Hemp seeds—Sometimes called hemp hearts, hemp seeds look like small split lentils that are mostly cream colored with some greens. They are soft and taste mildly nutty. They're a good source of omega-3s, and a three-tablespoon serving is a good source of protein, folate, magnesium, phosphorus, manganese, and B-vitamins. Try them on top of salads, avocado toast, porridges, or in smoothies, energy balls, or baked goods.

Pepitas—Shelled green pumpkin seeds, a serving of pepitas is one ounce, which works out to a little under a quarter cup. Pepitas are an excellent source of immunity-supportive zinc and a strong source of magnesium for quality sleep and strong bones, as well as providing iron, smaller amounts of other vitamins and minerals and antioxidants. Enjoy them in snacks, baked goods, and as a garnish.

Perilla seeds—Small, round, and light tan (raw) to shades of medium-brown (roasted), perilla seeds resemble tiny pebbles. They are pleasantly crunchy and taste nutty and mildly herbal, which makes sense since they are related to basil and mint. Perilla seeds are one of the best sources of plant-based omega-3 ALA, and one tablespoon offers nearly 4 grams of omega-3s. The daily recommended amount for adults is 1.1 to 1.6 grams per day to prevent a deficiency, and researchers think a higher amount may be more beneficial. They can be added to energy bites and cereal, sprinkled on rice bowls, or crushed and used in soups and sauces. Pre-crushed perilla "powder" or "flour" is available as are roasted and raw whole seeds.

Sesame seeds—Tiny flat seeds that are off-white when raw and tan when roasted. Black sesame seeds are a less common variety. They're a good source of fiber, which helps support regularity. Look for whole sesame seeds with their outer hulls intact because they will be higher in calcium. However, both hulled and unhulled sesame seeds will still be strong sources of magnesium, manganese, and zinc. Use them as a garnish, in dipping sauces, or as part of baked goods.

Beans

The MIND diet recommends eating beans, a kind of legume, four times a week or more. Beans are rich in plant protein, fiber, B vitamins, iron, potassium, and additional essential minerals. In addition to being nutrient-dense, they are low in total and saturated fat.

Diets higher in beans have been shown to slow cognitive decline. A study of more than 2,000 Swedish older adults aged 60 years and up showed that healthy diets that include beans provide neuroprotection. The same trend was found in a study of Taiwanese adults aged 65 years and up.

In addition to their contributions to brain health, beans belong in a healthy diet for their broad nutrition and health benefits. Beans have been positively associated with longevity in a cross-cultural study looking at food intake of adults aged 70 years and up from multiple cultures. This study found that for every 20 grams of beans eaten, the risk of mortality went down by 7 percent. Therefore, a Half cup serving of beans (85 grams) could reduce the risk of all-cause mortality by 30 percent.

Beans are also low-glycemic, slow-digesting carbohydrate foods, making them ideal for even blood sugar levels, and diabetes prevention and management. Their fiber and potassium are heart-healthy, and beans have been proven to improve cholesterol levels in people with heart disease. Last but not least, high fiber foods—and beans definitely qualify—are identified as probable protectors against colon and rectal cancer by the World Cancer Research Fund International and the American Institute for Cancer Research.

Beans are in a family of foods that includes healthy choices such as lentils, peas, and peanuts. The top five beans eaten in the United States are pinto beans, which account for about half of all beans grown and eaten domestically, navy beans, black beans, chickpeas, and Great Northern beans. Generally speaking, beans are an excellent source of folate and provide manganese, magnesium, iron, plant protein, fiber, potassium, and other important nutrients.

Both plant protein and plant iron are more efficiently absorbed when eaten together with animal protein such as Pacific cod, Alaskan salmon, or skinless chicken. Vitamin C from berries or vegetables also improves nutrient absorption. Combining these foods pulls even more nutrition out of beans.

All Forms Matter

Beans are available in fresh, dried, frozen, and canned forms. Cooked beans are available in BPA-free cans, as well as aseptic cartons, which are always BPA-free. For these kinds of packaged beans, drain and rinse them to remove about 40 percent of the sodium. For dried beans, the process requires some time, but is otherwise very simple: sort, rinse, soak, and cook (alternatively, skip the soak and cook low and slow for a longer period of time).

Dried beans are more affordable and closer to their natural state. They love moisture, low temperatures, and can stand up to long cooking times, making them ideal for slow-cooker dishes. Most dried beans need at least an hour to fully cook, though cranberry beans and great northern beans only need 45 to 60 minutes. Pink beans need about an hour. Black beans and small red beans need an hour to an hour and a half. The longest cooking beans need anywhere from an hour and a half to two hours, including dark red and light red kidney beans, navy beans, and pinto beans.

Get to Know Beans

Black beans—these get their deep dark color from anthocyanins, the same antioxidants that make blueberries blue. They are an excellent source of fiber, folate, iron, and magnesium. Black beans are commonly used in Caribbean, Central American, and South American recipes, and work well in salads, veggie burgers, and pureed into dips and soups. Cooking time: 60 to 90 minutes.

Cranberry beans—they are medium in size, oval in shape, and tan in color, streaked with cranberry red lines that disappear with cooking. They have a creamy texture and chestnut-like flavor, and are a favorite in northern Italy and Spain. They're also known as Roman beans. Cooking time: 45 to 60 minutes.

Green soybeans—refers to young green soybeans, sometimes referred to as máodòu (Taiwanese) or edamame (Japanese). They are rarely sold fresh and are most often found frozen. If found fresh, they should be kept dry, in a perforated plastic bag, and refrigerated for four to five days. Green soybeans contain all nine essential amino acids, making them an excellent vegetarian protein source. They are also a good source of vitamin A, calcium, and iron.

Fava beans—most often enjoyed fresh versus dried, fava beans should be in pods that are firm without too many markings. Pods should be heavy. They'll stay fresh for five to seven days in the refrigerator. They're an excellent source of fiber and folate, and can be enjoyed in hummus, soups, salads, or lightly sautéed with mushrooms for a delightful spring side dish.

Great northern beans—medium in size and oval in shape with a delicate and thin white skin, they have a mild, light flavor, making them a good choice for someone new to beans. Great northern beans are often used in French and Mediterranean cuisine. They are smaller than cannellinis and are versatile: they can be used in salads, soups, stews, and purees. Cooking time: 45 to 60 minutes.

Red kidney beans—Kidney beans are relatively large, and as the name suggests, kidney-shaped. The red variety have a deep red, glossy skin and a firm texture that withstands long cooking times, making them a smart choice for slow-cooking dishes such as soups and chilis. Cooking time: 90 to 120 minutes.

Light red kidney beans—just like dark red kidney beans, except the skin is a glossy light red to pink hue. The light red variety are popular in Caribbean, Portuguese, and Spanish dishes. Both dark red and light red kidney beans can be used in Louisiana red beans and rice. Cooking time: 90 to 120 minutes.

Lima beans—popular in Aztec and Inca cultures, lima beans are often in dried or canned forms. They are high in fiber and folate, and a good source of potassium and plant protein.

Navy beans—so called because they were a US Navy diet staple. They are small, white, oval-shaped beans with a mild and delicate flavor. Used in Boston baked beans, navy beans also work well in chilis, soups, and stews. They are rich in folate and fiber. Cooking time: 90 to 120 minutes.

Pink beans—a small, pink, oval-shaped bean that is healthfully prepared in a popular Caribbean dish made with sofrito (a mixture of tomato, bell pepper, onions, and garlic), with no added fat. Cooking time: 60 minutes.

Pinto beans—medium, oval-shaped beans with mottled beige and brown skin similar to cranberry beans; and like cranberry beans, the streaks on dried pinto beans disappear during cooking. Pinto beans are very common and popular in the Americas and are used in Mexican refried beans, but a lighter way to enjoy them is in a side dish with diced red bell peppers, extra-virgin olive oil, lemon juice, red onion, and fresh pepper. Cooking time: 90 to 120 minutes.

Small red beans—as their name implies, they are small and red. They're oval in shape, softer and with a more delicate flavor than red kidney beans. They're often eaten with rice in Caribbean dishes. Cooking time: 60 to 90 minutes.

Berries

Berries are specifically included in the MIND diet, even though fruit in general is not. This doesn't mean you should avoid other fruit, a naturally healthy food. The takeaway is to prioritize including berries in your diet at least twice a week for brain health. Eating them more often and enjoying a variety of other fruit in addition to berries is still a good goal. But for brain health in particular, berries have shown promise for both short- and long-term cognitive benefits. Research suggests antioxidants in berries (anthocyanins) improve memory, and sometimes improve attention, psychomotor speed, and executive function, according to a 2021 meta-analysis of randomized-controlled trials.[27]

Short-term experimental studies have shown that berries improve cognition, perhaps because berries are high in flavonoids, especially the kind called anthocyanidins, which have antioxidant and anti-inflammatory functions. Multiple animal studies have found that adding blueberries or strawberries to their diets reduced age-related declines in neural signaling and cognitive skills. In fact, in older rats, neuronal and cognitive aging was reversed. And these findings are supported by clinical research in humans.

In a study of older men with early cognitive impairments, adding blueberries or grape juice to their diets helped improve memory

---

27 S. Ahles, P. J. Joris, and J. Plat, "Effects of Berry Anthocyanins on Cognitive Performance, Vascular Function, and Cardiometabolic Risk Markers: A Systematic Review of Randomized Placebo-Controlled Intervention Studies in Humans," *International Journal of Molecular Sciences* 22, no. 12 (2021): 6482, https://doi.org/10.3390/ijms22126482.

abilities. A 2017 randomized controlled trial found that a mixed berry beverage improved working memory.[28]

A large, long-term study also points to the brain benefits of berries. Based on diet data that was collected over 21 years (1980–2001) from more than 16,000 women, a study in a subset of the Nurses' Health Study (NHS) found that total flavonoids, including anthocyanidins, can slow down the cognitive aging process by an average of up to two and a half years, and that berries were especially potent. Blueberries and strawberries were the most common sources of anthocyanidins in the diets of NHS participants.

People who ate blueberries once a week or more had better cognitive function, making them up to three and a half years younger than people who had a half cup or less per month. For strawberries, those who ate two or more servings per week were cognitively up to three years younger than those who had less than a half cup per week. A 2021 randomized clinical trial found that eating two cups of strawberries a day improved learning and memory,[29] and a 2019 observational study found that eating strawberries once a week or more reduced the risk of Alzheimer's by 34 percent.[30]

In the US, strawberries are the most popular berry, and may be a good place to start. But don't stop there. Enjoying a variety of berries will mean benefitting from a wider range of protective plant compounds, sometimes called phytonutrients or bioactives. Anthocyanidins and anthocyanins are widely found in foods that are naturally red, blue, and purple.

28 A. Nilsson et al., "Effects of a Mixed Berry Beverage on Cognitive Functions and Cardio-metabolic Risk Markers," *PloS One*12, no. 11 (2017): e0188173, https://doi.org/10.1371/journal.pone.0188173.

29 M. G. Miller et al., "Dietary Strawberry Improves Cognition in a Randomised, Double-Blind, Placebo-Controlled Trial in Older Adults," *British Journal of Nutrition* 126, no. 2 (2021):253–263, https://doi.org/10.1017/S0007114521000222.

30 Agarwal et al., "Association of Strawberries and Anthocyanidin Intake with Alzheimer's Dementia Risk," *Nutrients* 11, no. 12 (2019), https://doi.org/10.3390/nu11123060.

Common food sources of anthocyanidins and anthocyanins:[31]

- Blackberries
- Blueberries
- Cranberries
- Raspberries
- Red cabbage
- Red grapes
- Red, purple, and blueish leafy greens
- Red wine
- Strawberries

Common food sources of flavonoids in general:[32]

- Apples
- Cherries
- Chickpeas
- Dark chocolate
- Dried oregano
- Dried parsley
- Grapefruit
- Lemons
- Limes
- Oranges
- Onions
- Tea
- Wine

Total flavonoids are more important than any one source, but anthocyanidins in berries are capable of crossing the blood-brain barrier and finding their way to local brain regions used in learning and memory such as the hippocampus. More generally, many

---

31 Khoo et al., "Anthocyanidins and Anthocyanins," *Food and Nutrition Research* 61, no. 1 (2017): 1361779, doi: 10.1080/16546628.2017.1361779.

32 Janabi et al., "Flavonoid-Rich Foods (FRF)," *Iranian Journal of Basic Medical Science* 23, no. 2 (2022): 140–153, doi: 10.22038/IJBMS.2019.35125.8353.

flavonoids can help reduce inflammation in the brain and spinal cord. Flavonoid-rich foods can also activate certain receptors and pathways that are believed to enhance memory and cognition.

The MIND diet recommends eating berries twice a week. Blueberries and strawberries are widely available and popular. There are many additional berries to try, especially in the summer when a wide variety are in season, at peak quality, and usually most affordable. At times when fresh isn't available or convenient, frozen, canned, dried, and 100 percent juice forms are options.

Most berries are highly perishable and should be stored in the refrigerator without anything heavy on top, which can lead to bruising and spoilage. Wash just before using.

Fall Berries

Barbados cherries—native to the West Indies, Central and South America, these cherries grow well in tropical and subtropical areas, including Florida. They're an excellent source of vitamins A and C. Choose firm, red cherries with the stems still attached. They'll last in the refrigerator for up to five days, or can be frozen for six months.

Black crowberries—a cold-loving berry, these small, black berries grow in Alaska, Canada, Newfoundland, and Greenland, and are popular in northern Europe. They are packed with antioxidants, manganese, and vitamin C. Choosing crowberries is similar to choosing good blueberries. Look for firm, plump, dry berries that are dusty blue to black. They'll last up to two weeks in the refrigerator.

Cape gooseberry—they get their name from a light tan to brown papery "cape" that surrounds them and makes them look a little like tomatillos (see Vegetables). They are green when young, but ripen to yellow. They are tart and have a similar texture to cherries. They're an excellent source of vitamins A and C, potassium, copper, and fiber. Choose brightly colored gooseberries with dry capes, though the capes are sometimes removed before shipping. They can be stored in the refrigerator for up to a week.

Cranberries–a holiday favorite, cranberries are native to North America and are called cranberries because the flowers look like cranes. Cranberries are a good source of vitamin C and fiber and are quite hardy; they can be refrigerated for up to two months. Look for firm cranberries that aren't shriveled or browning.

Huckleberry–a Midwest favorite that can be interchanged easily with blueberries, huckleberries even resemble blueberries. The huckleberry is wild and native to North America, and also goes by the names bilberry, wineberry, and dyeberry. Choose smooth berries without mold. Huckleberries are an excellent source of vitamin C and antioxidants, and are best stored frozen after washing and drying.

Pomegranate–see Winter.

Winter Berries

Pomegranate–an antioxidant powerhouse, each pomegranate contains hundreds of seeds, called arils, surrounded by red flesh, both of which are edible. Pomegranates are an excellent source of fiber, vitamins C and K, potassium, folate, and copper. Choose pomegranates that are plump, round, and heavy for their size. They can be stored in a cool, dry area for a month, or in the refrigerator for up to two months.

Red currants–due to their tart flavor, red currants are commonly used in jams and pie fillings, though healthier ways to include them in the diet are in smoothies or in no-sugar-added sauces for chicken. They're an excellent source of vitamin C and antioxidants, and can be stored unwashed in the refrigerator for up to a week. Choose brightly colored berries without mold or soft spots.

Spring Berries

Barbados cherries–see Fall.

Lychee–sometimes spelled litchi, this member of the soapberry family has roots in China that go back more than 2,000 years. They resemble large raspberries, but their skin is rough and inedible. The flesh inside is white with a single large seed. Choose fruit that is heavy for its size, and know that brown patches mean that the fruit inside will be sweeter. They can be refrigerated inside a plastic bag for up to 10 days. Lychee are an excellent source of vitamin C.

Strawberries—these popular berries are covered in about 200 tiny seeds per berry, and are rich in vitamin C and folate. They should be shiny, firm, and bright red with fresh green caps. Look out for shriveled or mushy berries. They can be stored in the refrigerator unwashed for one to three days. They are most popular berry in the United States.

Summer Berries

Barbados cherries—see Fall.

Black crowberry—see Fall.

Black currants—these berries look like small, round, dark grapes, though they are not nearly as sweet. Because of their tartness, they are usually used in jellies and jams, and could also be used in smoothies and sauces. They are an excellent source of vitamin C, fiber, potassium, and manganese. Look for dry, firm, round currants, and stay vigilant for signs of moldy or crushed berries. Sort through them at home, and store the good berries in the refrigerator, unwashed, for up to a week. They can also be stored frozen for up to a year.

Blackberries—sometimes mistaken for black raspberries, the difference is that they have a solid center (raspberries are hollow). They're an excellent source of vitamin C and fiber, and can be stored, unwashed, for three to six days.

Blueberries—a good source of vitamin C and fiber, blueberries are highly researched due to their high antioxidant activity. Look for firm, plump, dry blueberries with a dusty blue color. They can be stored in the refrigerator for up to two weeks.

Boysenberries–a hybrid of raspberries and blackberries, boysenberries are reddish-purple. They're an excellent source of fiber, folate, manganese, and vitamin K. Look for shiny, plump, firm berries, and avoid any berries that look bruised or wet. Sort through them at home to remove any moldy berries, then refrigerate, unwashed, for up to a week.

Cherries–a summertime favorite, cherries are a good source of vitamin C and potassium. Look for firm, red cherries with good color and stems still attached. They'll last in the refrigerator for up to 10 days.

Sour cherries–more tart than the common cherry, sour cherries are an excellent source of vitamins A, C, and fiber, and can be stored, unwashed, for two to three days in the refrigerator. They can also be rinsed, deseeded, and frozen for later use. Look for clean, bright, shiny, plump berries without blemishes. They can be enjoyed fresh, but for those that don't prefer the tart flavor on its own, it can be balanced by adding to whole grain dishes.

Elderberries–these small, dark berries are an excellent source of fiber, vitamins A, C, and B6, and they provide vitamin E, copper, and iron too. Look for firm berries with rich, dark color. Sort out any mushy berries at home and store the good, unwashed berries in the refrigerator for up to a week.

Loganberries–named after a judge named Logan in Santa Cruz who grew them in his backyard in the late 19th century, loganberries should be shiny, plump, firm, and red. They can be stored in the refrigerator for up to a week, unwashed. Loganberries are rich in vitamin C, fiber, and manganese. They also provide vitamin K and folate.

Longan–similar to lychee but smaller and with a smoother skin that is tan instead of red, longan also belongs to the soapberry family. They're an excellent source of vitamin C and can be stored in plastic bags in the refrigerator for up to a week. Look for longans with an intense tan color, which indicates they are ripe. They should be firm and free of bruising or blemishes.

Lychee—see Spring.

Mulberries—they resemble and can easily be substituted for blackberries. They are an excellent source of vitamin C and manganese, and also provide vitamin K and iron. Look for mulberries that are shiny, plump, and firm. Avoid any berries that are bruised or wet. They can be stored, unwashed, in the refrigerator for up to a week.

Omija berries—native to Korea, China, Japan, and Russia, and now cultivated in Europe and North America, omija are small red berries with a strong flavor and therefore not commonly consumed raw. They can be found dried, powdered, in tea blends, and extracts. Omija are known as the "five flavor fruit" because they offer a unique medley of salty, sweet, sour, pungent, and bitter flavors all at once. They are used in traditional Chinese medicine, and a 2017 in vitro study using cell samples (vs. live subjects) suggests they may inhibit the formation of amyloid plaques in the brain.[33]

Strawberries—see Spring.

Raspberries—while commonly red, raspberries can be black, purple, and even golden in color. They are rich in vitamin C and fiber, and can be stored unwashed in the refrigerator for a day or two. Look for dry, plump, and firm raspberries. Avoid wet or moldy berries.

Poultry

The MIND diet recommends eating poultry twice a week, specifically noting that it should not be fried. In addition to providing a healthy protein to the diet, lean poultry is a source of vitamin B12, an essential nutrient that has received a great amount of attention in scientific literature for its role in brain health.

---

[33] Zhang et al., "The Influence of Schisandrin B on a Model of Alzheimer's Disease," *Journal of Toxicology and Environmental Health* 80, no. 22 (2017).

Poultry provides high-quality protein that includes all of the essential amino acids, as well as iron and zinc, in forms that the body can readily absorb them (i.e., improves their bioavailability). Pairing poultry with plant foods that contain iron and zinc also helps make those nutrients more bioavailable.

While it is a healthy alternative to red meat, it is not an everyday food in the MIND diet. This is similar to its position in the plant-based Mediterranean and DASH diet patterns. The American Heart Association recommends poultry without the skin, baked or grilled, twice a week.

The most common poultry you'll find at the grocery store are chicken and turkey. Light meat (breast meat) is generally leaner than dark meat (thighs), and many cuts are available already skinless.

However, skin-on, bone-in, or whole birds are often more affordable, and just require a little extra prep time to remove skin and trim visible fat before eating. For ground chicken and turkey, choose at least 90 to 95 percent lean options.

For the time-pressed, most grocers offer whole rotisserie chicken that is hot, fully cooked, and ready to go. Some offer roasted turkey as well. A few cautions though: Seek out no-salt-added items, and avoid the options with words like "savory" or "juicy," which can be code for "pumped with added salt." At home, remove the skin and visible fat.

Another option some grocers offer is plain (versatile) grilled chicken in the refrigerated case that can be tossed into salads, stir-fry dishes, soups, and stews. Keep in mind that the tradeoff for the convenience of letting someone else do the cooking for you is less control over food safety practices, so only buy from food providers you trust to minimize risk.

At home, refrigerate raw poultry in the coldest area of the refrigerator, which is normally on the bottom shelf, in the back, farthest from the door. It can be stored here for up to two days, or frozen for up to two months. Cooked poultry can be refrigerated for up to three days, or frozen for up to one month.

Fish

The MIND diet includes at least one fish meal a week that is not fried, which is simpler than the several fish meals per week required by the Mediterranean diet. The MIND diet recommends just one serving per week because the research did not show additional brain health benefits with higher levels of intake. Eating fish and omega-3 fats has been associated with lower risk of Alzheimer's disease and stroke. Fish is a direct source of omega-3s, including docosapentaenoic acid (DHA), which is especially important for cognitive development and a normally functioning brain.

Small studies have shown a modest cognitive benefit with one fish meal a week. Large-scale population studies in older populations in the United States (Chicago Health and Aging Project, or CHAP), the Netherlands (Rotterdam Study), and France (PAQUID study) have also shown that fish intake lowers the risk of Alzheimer's disease.

A large study of older Chicago residents explored the relationship between fish, omega-3s, and cognitive decline. They studied 3,718 adults aged 65 years and older who were part of CHAP over a period of six years. After six years, people eating fish once or twice a week slowed down their cognitive aging by 10 to 13 percent per year, or the equivalent to being three to four years younger.

Even though one fish meal per week is enough to lower the risk of dementia, there may be other reasons to enjoy fish more often for heart health and as a lean protein choice. A research review of nine population studies found that eating fish more often reduced the risk of stroke in a dose-response manner (that is, more fish, more benefits). The *Dietary Guidelines for Americans 2020–2025* recommends two fish meals per week, or about eight ounces for the week.

Is Fried Fish OK?

It's common knowledge that frying is not the healthiest way to prepare a meal, but sometimes the benefits of eating a healthy food outweigh the risks (case in point, see the section below on mercury in fish). However, in the case of frying, that does not seem to be the case. Frying reduces omega-3 fat levels and increases saturated fat intake. In a large study, the Cardiovascular Health Study (CHS), eating fish only reduced the risk of Alzheimer's disease if it was fatty fish that was not fried. There was no such benefit seen with fried fish. In another large study, the Women's Health Initiative Observational Study, women who ate five (or more) servings of fish per week cut their risk of heart failure by 30 percent, but only if it was baked or broiled fish. In fact, in the same study, women who ate fried fish one (or more) times per week increased their risk of heart failure by 50 percent.

SHOULD YOU BE WORRIED ABOUT MERCURY IN FISH?

Seafood is one of the healthiest foods around, but fish can also be a source of mercury, a known neurotoxin. Mercury can build up in a pregnant woman's body to levels that can put the developing child at risk for poor cognitive performance in attention, fine motor tests, language, visual-spatial skills, and verbal memory.

Mercury also builds up in fish over a time, from both natural and industrial sources in the environment. Thus, longer-living larger fish like tilefish, swordfish, shark, and king mackerel will be higher in mercury than, say, scallops, salmon, shrimp, anchovies, or freshwater trout, which are smaller and shorter living.

Pregnant women and young children are cautioned by the FDA to avoid certain fish because of their mercury content and should seek out low-mercury options. It can be helpful to think of the acronym TSSK to remember the higher mercury fish listed earlier; appropriately, the acronym itself sounds like a warning or disapproval. However, for middle-aged and older men and women, health experts agree that the benefits far outweigh the risks.

Until 2016, very little was known about how eating seafood affected the brain's level of mercury and disease markers for dementia. A study published in the *Journal of the American Medical Association*, and led by MIND diet researcher Dr. Morris, asked two questions: 1) Did eating seafood mean higher levels of mercury in the brain? and 2) How was seafood intake or brain mercury associated with brain diseases, if at all?

The study population was a cross section of people from the Memory and Aging Project (MAP) in Chicago, who passed away between 2004 and 2013. Diet information was collected regularly as part of the MAP study, and out of 554 deceased participants, about half (48.4 percent) had brain autopsies. Not surprisingly, the researchers found that eating more seafood did indeed lead to higher levels of mercury in the brain. Surprisingly, when it came to Alzheimer's disease, eating more than one seafood meal per week was associated with healthier brains even with higher levels of mercury in the brain. The neuritic plaques and tangles were more sparse in the fish eaters than those who didn't eat fish, who tended to have more severe and widespread tangles and a higher concentration of brain plaques.

Study participants ate an average of one to three fish meals per week, and according to the National Marine Fisheries Service, the top 10 most commonly consumed fish in the United States already have low-to-moderate levels of mercury (shrimp, salmon, canned tuna, tilapia, pollock, pangasius, cod, catfish, crab, and clams). Therefore, it's hard to say whether these results would hold true if the study participants had eaten higher-mercury fish, more frequent fish meals, or both.

The take-home message is that moderate fish intake is a healthy choice for cognitive health. It is already well-established as a nutritious protein for heart health, diabetes, general health, and longevity. This study adds to the positive news by linking moderate fish intake with lower signs of Alzheimer's disease, even with higher brain levels of mercury that go up as fish intake goes up.

Finding Fresh Fish

Choosing fresh fish is simple with a few key tips. For whole fish, look for red gills (not brown), shiny metallic skin, and clear, bright eyes, both of which fade or dull when a fish has passed its peak. Gently press into the flesh of the fish and see how quickly the indentation disappears. Fresh fish has firm and resilient flesh without any gaps between layers. If there is liquid on the fish, it should run clear and not milky, which is an early sign of rotting. Lastly, fish should smell like clean ocean water (saltwater fish) or a clean pond (freshwater fish), but never pungent or "fishy."

Starter Seafood

If seafood isn't yet a regular part of your diet or you aren't sure it's your favorite, try starting with a mild, flaky white fish such as Pacific cod or halibut. These fish are buttery and delicate, and pick up the flavors they're cooked with, making them perfect for a gentle introduction to the wide world of seafood. Another great option is to mash anchovies and incorporate them into pasta sauces, which adds savory flavor without adding a fishy taste.

Frozen and canned fish are conveniently available year-round when fresh fish isn't practical.

Easy Swaps

What a recipe calls for and what's available at your local store may not always match up. Check out the lists below to see what types of fish are interchangeable.

White, lean, flaky fish: Atlantic croaker, black sea bass, branzino (aka European sea bass), flounder, rainbow smelt, red snapper, tilapia, rainbow trout, weakfish (sea trout), whiting

White, lean, firm fish: Alaska pollock, catfish, grouper, haddock, Pacific cod, Pacific halibut, Pacific rockfish, Pacific sand dab and sole, striped bass (wild and hybrid), swordfish

White, firm, oily fish: Atlantic shad, Albacore tuna, California white sea bass, Chilean sea bass, cobia, lake trout, lake whitefish, Pacific escolar, Pacific sablefish, white sturgeon

Medium and oily fish: Amberjack, Arctic char, Hawaiian kampachi, mahi mahi, paddlefish, pompano, salmon (coho or sockeye), wahoo

Dark and oily fish: Anchovies, blue fin tuna, grey mullet, herring (Atlantic, Boston, or king), salmon (farmed or king/chinook), sardines, kkipjack, tuna

Sustainable Seafood

There are a number of ways to identify sustainably harvested (for farmed) and caught (for wild) fish. There is some confusion over wild versus farmed fish and what is more environmentally friendly. Unfortunately, there is no simple rule about what's better. There are damaging practices in both farmed and wild caught seafood. Sometimes the issue is that the population of the fish species is low, other times it may be that the way it's caught catches and kills other species, or the way it's farmed breeds disease and pollutes the water. These are just a few of the concerns.

It's a lot to keep track of, but that's exactly what credible scientific organizations such as the The Safina Center in New York and Monterey Bay Aquarium in California do. They provide good general recommendations, and for additional assurances, there are trustworthy third-party certifications given by the Marine Stewardship Council (for wild fish) and Aquaculture Stewardship Council (for farmed fish). This is an evolving issue, and as fish populations grow stronger or fish are caught or grown in more responsible ways, some fish may move from the "do not eat" to the "go ahead and enjoy" category.

Olive Oil

Similar to the Mediterranean diet, the MIND diet uses olive oil as its main fat. Olive oil boasts approximately 230 antioxidants and polyphenols. While the whole is more than its parts, it's possible that one such part, oleocanthal, has an especially protective role in brain health. Oleocanthal is one of hundreds of natural phenolic compounds in extra-virgin olive oil with antioxidant and anti-inflammatory properties. In an animal study published in *ACS Chemical Neuroscience*, oleocanthal helped shuttle abnormal proteins (beta-amyloid) out of the brain. The accumulation of beta-amyloid proteins form plaques that eventually disrupt nerve cell function, leading to the death of the affected brain cells, which is believed to be culprit in Alzheimer's disease. Oleocanthal boosted production of proteins and enzymes that are essential to removing beta-amyloid from the brain. In a sub-study of the larger PREDIMED trial, people eating diets supplemented with olive oil were associated with better immediate and delayed forms of verbal memory.

The MIND diet has no restriction on total fat and recommends olive oil as the main source of fat, especially in place of solid fats like butter, stick margarine, lard, and coconut oil. In the Mediterranean diet, it's not uncommon to consume 2 to 3 tablespoons per day, and the PREDIMED study recommends about 4 tablespoons of olive oil per day.

Extra-virgin olive oil, which is simply pressed olives, is special because it provides vitamins E and K, plus protective polyphenols. The most important things to know are that extra-virgin olive oil isn't for cooking, and all olive oil should come in dark or opaque containers to preserve the quality of the oil, as it breaks down with heat and light.

Extra-virgin olive oil is a finishing oil and should be enjoyed in salad dressings and on top of soups, toasts, and other dishes. It's not meant to be heated to high temperatures, which destroys the complex flavor that comes from the polyphenols and other phytonutrients; these, in turn, are what drive a premium price. Use regular olive oil for cooking, but even then, use it for low-heat cooking due to its relatively low smoke point (the temperature at which the oil begins to smoke and degrade into damaging free radicals). Going above the smoke point causes damage to the oil that in turn can make it unhealthy to consume. For high-heat cooking, try a grapeseed oil, or a blend of olive oil with another vegetable oil.

Heat and light, as well as water and air, are enemies to all cooking oils. Olive oil, with its many phytonutrients, is no different. Look for containers that are dark glass, tin, or even clear glass, but then mostly covered with a label or box to protect the oil and its polyphenols from going bad too quickly. Store it in a cool, dark place away from the stove. It can be refrigerated, but it's not recommended, especially for higher-quality olive oils. Buy the right size of olive oil that will be used in a couple of months. This may mean buying smaller containers of olive oil to ensure it's being used at its best.

Find Good-Quality Olive Oil

Look for a harvest date. Good producers will include a date on the olive oil bottle indicating when the olives were harvested. Try to pick out an oil that's within a year of its harvest. The closer to the harvest date the better. Northern hemisphere olives (e.g., from California, Spain, Italy, Greece) are usually harvested in November to December, and southern hemisphere olives (e.g., from Argentina, Australia, Chile, Peru) are typically harvested in May to June. Depending on the time it takes to process and bottle the oil, choosing olive oils closer to their harvest date may mean looking for California olive oil earlier in the year, and Australian olive oil in the second half of the year. The harvest date is not a "best by" date, which is often two years from the time the bottle was filled, not when the olives were harvested or processed.

Taste for freshness. Olive oil should taste vegetal or "green," slightly bitter, and have a peppery kick you can feel at the back of your throat when swallowing (this is a sign of healthy polyphenols in the oil, and a cough is not an uncommon first reaction). A quality olive oil can have fruity notes that range from grassy to apple to green banana and artichoke. It should not taste musty, metallic, or buttery, nor should it taste or smell like wine or vinegar.

Look for quality assurances. Recently, olive oil fraud has become an issue as manufacturers mix olive oil with colorings, flavors, and less expensive oils. In response to the questions about olive oil authenticity, some industry standards have emerged from the California Olive Oil Council (COOC) and the Australian Olive Oil Association (AOOA), which offer quality seals to identify olive oils that meet higher-quality standards than the minimal USDA ones.

A World of Flavors and Acidity

Olive oils are graded by acidity level, and the best ones are cold-pressed, which is a chemical-free process that simply involves pressure and results in a naturally low level of acidity. This is the way in which extra-virgin olive oil is made, resulting in a one-percent acidity oil. It can be dark green to light champagne in color, with the darker-color oils offering the most intense olive flavors.

Italian olive oil tends to be dark green and has an herbal and grassy scent and flavor. Greek olive oil also tends to be green and is marked by strong flavors and aromas. Spain is one of the world's largest olive oil producers, and their olive oil commonly appears golden yellow and tastes both fruity and nutty. In contrast, French olive oil tends to be pale and mild in flavor. California olive oil also tends to be light in color and flavor, but with a fruitier taste. Any of these can be of extra-virgin quality.

Virgin olive oil is also a first-press oil, but the level of acidity is slightly higher in the 1 to 3 percent range. Oils simply labeled as "olive oil" could be a mix of refined olive oil and virgin or extra-virgin olive oil. It used to be called "pure" olive oil. Light olive oil is a refined olive oil that is light in flavor and color, not calories. Light olive oil has a higher smoke point than regular olive oil, so it's better for low- and medium-heat cooking.

Wine

Including alcohol in a therapeutic diet is complicated and ultimately an individual choice, perhaps made in collaboration with your personal health care team. In fact, the 2023 MIND trial excluded alcohol for safety reasons. It's important to remember that it's entirely possible to reach therapeutic levels of the MIND diet without drinking wine. Generally, people who do not already drink wine should not start because they are following the MIND diet, and those who do drink should consume no more than 5 ounces a day.

The MIND diet includes a 5-ounce glass of wine a day, no more, no less. This comes from the Mediterranean diet influence. For example, wine, a polyphenol-rich food, is associated with better cognitive function in a recent sub-study of the larger PREDIMED trial (Spain). In the sub-study of 447 older men and women ages 55 to 80 years, those who drank wine scored better on the mini–mental state exam, a 30-point set of questions that test a range of everyday mental skills, from being able to identify the correct year, spell a word backward, remember a series of words mentioned earlier, repeat phrases, and more. It's important to note that this study was done in Spain, where wine is part of the lifestyle and potentially more likely to be consumed in moderation and as part of meals. Findings from one country don't always translate to another due to cultural differences.

While observational studies suggest moderate alcohol intake reduces the risk of Alzheimer's disease, they also point to high intakes increasing the risk. A review on alcohol, dementia, and pre-dementia suggests that the protective effects of moderate alcohol intake, such as the one glass of wine a day in the MIND diet, are more promising in people without the common genetic marker for Alzheimer's disease, APOE-e4.[34] It's also more promising for wine compared to other types of alcohol. This same paper concludes that there are no signs light drinking would be harmful to cognition and dementia. However, a 2023 report from the World Health Organization that was focused on cancer prevention (vs. brain health or cardiovascular health) declared that there is no safe amount of alcohol. They specified that it was the alcohol, not any specific beverage, that did the harm. Therefore, nonalcoholic wines, cooked wines, and wine-based vinegars may confer benefits without the risk of consuming alcohol.

Red wine contains resveratrol and other polyphenols, which are antioxidants and anti-inflammatory. As potent antioxidants, they may help, in conjunction with a diet rich in polyphenols, to reduce and protect against the formation of the beta-amyloid plaques that come with Alzheimer's disease. Interestingly, a study of alcohol-free wine, an excellent source of antioxidants, found that it was effective in increasing antioxidant activity.

A serving size is five ounces (be mindful, as today's glassware often holds multiple servings). When it comes to the best way to incorporate wine with food, the first rule to live by is to drink according to your preferences, and let your own palate and budget be your guide. Other than that, there are a few guiding principles of how to pair food and wine, but these are just suggestions. Below are some recommendations for wines that generally pair well with the brain-healthy foods in the MIND diet.

Again, ultimately, drinking wine is a personal choice that may be important for cultural reasons, and there are ways to thrive both with and without it.

---

34   F. Panza et al., "Alcohol Consumption in Mild Cognitive Impairment and Dementia," *International Journal of Geriatric Psychiatry* 27, no. 12 (2012): 1218–1238.

Vegetables—Raw vegetables, such as those in a crudités platter, go well with white wines such as chardonnay, pinot blanc, and chenin blanc. Asparagus goes great with white wines such as sauvignon blanc and dry Riesling. Stir fry vegetables with east Asian flavor (e.g. soy, rice vinegar, chili) is complemented by slightly sweet German Rieslings.

Nuts—The savory-rich flavors and mouthfeel of heart-healthy fats from nuts go well with dry (brut) sparkling wines and champagne. Nuts can also stand up to the richness of a fortified wine such as port.

Beans—Pairing wine with beans is more about what kind of bean is used and how it is prepared. Generally, mild white beans will work with white wines, and headier and hardier beans that may be used in chilis will work better with reds. Summer recipes may work best with chardonnay or rosé, and richer recipes may work better with reds.

Berries—It's true: strawberries and champagne are a match made in heaven. Generally, berries pair well with sparkling wines—from dry to semi-dry, as well as sweeter white wines like Riesling and muscat. To try something a little different, pair berries with a light red wine like zinfandel.

Poultry—Chicken is versatile, and so are the wines that pair with it, from white wines like chardonnay, vin gris, Riesling, and chenin blanc to lighter reds like merlot and pinot noir. Chicken dishes made with savory tomatoes and mushrooms may work best with a light red wine; chicken made with brighter flavors such as ginger, garlic, or lemon may work best with white wines. A picnic-worthy chicken salad would work nicely with slightly sweeter white wines such as Riesling or gewürztraminer. Turkey pairs nicely with red wines such as merlot and zinfandel, and with white wines such as chardonnay.

Fish—Tuna goes well with white wine, such as sauvignon blanc. The richness of salmon pairs well with pinot noir as well as some white wines, from pinot gris to sauvignon blanc. The fresh, clean flavors of sashimi generally pair well with dry sparkling wine, dry

Riesling, or a soft red like pinot noir or beaujolais. However, the wines that work best with specific types of sushi may vary.

Whole grains—Whole grain pasta salad goes well with white wines such as sauvignon blanc and dry Rieslings. If the pasta is prepared with tomato sauce, a light red wine may work better, such as a zinfandel.

Olive oil—Similar to nuts, the velvety mouthfeel of heart-healthy fats from olive oil goes well with dry (brut) sparkling wines and champagne.

By the glass—If, instead, you are starting with a bottle of wine and are looking for inspiration on what to make for dinner that may go well with it, here are a few guidelines.

WINE COLOR	TYPES OF FISH
White	*Champagne* for savory foods *Sauvignon blanc* for tart dressings and sauces (citrus, vinegar) *Gruner veltliner* with herbs *Pinot grigio* with light dishes *Chardonnay* with fatty fish or fish in a rich sauce Slightly sweet *Riesling* with sweet and spicy dishes such as Asian dishes (also applies to *gewürztraminers* and *vouvrays*) *Moscato d'asti* for fruit desserts
Rosé/Reds	*Rosé champagne* for hors d'oeuvres and dinner, it's versatile *Pinot noir* with earthy flavors like mushrooms and bitter vegetables *Malbec* and spicy dishes as it's bold enough to withstand strong flavors *Syrah* for spicy dishes

Finally, remember that these are broad guidelines, and that your preferences may be very different. In addition, if dining out, a sommelier can share more specific recommendations for wine pairings and menu items.

CHAPTER 4

BRAIN-HARMING FOODS

The MIND diet's five types of brain-harming foods are red meat, butter and stick margarine, whole-fat cheese, pastries and sweets, and fried fast foods. Limiting these foods was part of the diet that led to better cognitive aging and reduced the risk of Alzheimer's disease in the MIND studies. The MIND researchers note that these are all foods that increase the intake of saturated and trans fats in proportion to unsaturated fats, which leads to blood-brain barrier problems and increases beta-amyloid plaque. In addition, two of the food groups—pastries and sweets and fried fast food—provide little nutrition, and most generally healthy diets recommend limiting them.

The MIND diet advice to avoid saturated fat agrees with the recent *Dietary Guidelines for Americans 2020–2025*, which recommends limiting saturated fat to less than 10 percent of total calories (22 grams or less in a 2000-calorie diet). The human body makes all the saturated fat it needs, which means there is zero biological need to have any saturated fat in the diet. According to the government report, there is strong and consistent evidence that replacing saturated fat with unsaturated fat—especially the polyunsaturated type—lowers LDL (bad) cholesterol and heart attacks. Similar evidence exists for the benefits of eating monounsaturated fats such as olive oil and nuts instead of saturated fat from foods like butter, margarine, beef, whole-fat cheese, sweets, and fried fast food.

Current research suggests saturated fat may be neutral when it comes to heart disease, usually when it replaces a refined carbohydrate. What we do know is that countless studies show that replacing saturated fat with polyunsaturated fat reduces heart disease risk. In addition, there are several studies in the area of cognitive decline and Alzheimer's disease suggesting an increased risk coming from too much saturated fat in the diet. Regardless of whether saturated fat is neutral instead of harmful, there are healthier fats to include in the diet. Unsaturated fats are found in nuts, fish, olive oil, and other plant oils that are liquid at room temperature.

Though the primary goal is to improve the quality of fat intake, limiting many of these foods will also reduce added sugars. Many studies point to excessive intake of added sugars being pro-inflammatory and that sugary foods such as sodas are associated with poorer cognitive function.

Five Food Groups to Limit

Red Meat

Red meat includes beef, lamb, duck, and pork. They may be in meat products such as hamburgers, beef tacos and burritos, hot dogs, sausages, meatballs, meatloaf, and deli meats. It's best to limit the fattiest cuts of these meats due to their saturated fat content.

The MIND diet recommends limiting red meat to less than four times per week. The World Health Organization classified processed meat as a group 1 carcinogen in October 2015 (the same category as tobacco and asbestos), noting that evidence suggests red meat probably is too. Being designated as a "group 1 carcinogen" is the strongest rating, and means there is convincing evidence that the substance causes cancer.

The damaging effects are seen over many meals, days, weeks, and years. A 2015 study of Taiwanese adults aged 65 years and up found that typical Western eating patterns high in meat increased the risk of cognitive decline over eight years compared to a healthy diet that included vegetables, beans, fish, fruit, and legumes. Over the eight-year period, a Western dietary pattern nearly tripled the risk of cognitive decline. A multi-decade study of more than 120,000 men and women, conducted by Harvard researcher Frank Hu and his team, estimated that swapping out a serving of red meat each day with healthier protein options such as fish, poultry, nuts, beans, low-fat dairy, and whole grains could lower the risk of death by 7 to 19 percent.

If you don't already enjoy red meat, there's no reason to start. But if you do choose to eat red meat occasionally, follow these basic guidelines to do it in the healthier ways:

- **Choose the least processed meat possible.** That means choosing fresh cuts of meat versus processed meat like bacon, beef jerky, bologna, canned meat, ham, hot dogs, mortadella, pastrami, pepperoni, salami, and sausages. Many deli meats fall into this category, though sliced lunch meat that is simply cooked and sliced isn't considered processed, such as roast beef, turkey, and chicken.

- **Opt for grass-fed, organic meat.** It tends to be leaner and has a different nutrient profile due to the grass-based diet, including more carotenoids, vitamin E, potassium, iron, and zinc than conventional meat.

- **Look for fresh meat at the grocery store that is labeled as "lean," "extra lean," or "loin."** Choose cuts that are "choice" or "select" over fattier cuts labeled as "prime."

- **For ground meats, look for the lowest percentage of fat.** For example, "95 percent lean meat, 5 percent fat."

Beef—"extra lean" cuts of beef are eye round roast/steak, sirloin tip side steak, top round roast/steak, bottom round roast/steak, and top sirloin steak.

Bison—sirloin, rib eye, and top round cuts all have 2 grams of fat per serving.

Veal—leg, sirloin, and loin all have 3 grams or less fat per serving.

Pork—tenderloin has 2 grams fat per serving, and sirloin cuts have about 4 grams of fat per serving.

Lamb—lamb shank, loin, and shoulder have 6 grams of fat or less per serving.

Butter and Stick Margarine

The MIND diet recommends limiting butter and stick margarine to less than a tablespoon per day. Generally, any fat that is solid at room temperature has too much saturated fat to be included in the MIND diet, including the butter and stick margarine already mentioned, but also palm oil, coconut oil, beef tallow, lard, and shortening.

The MIND diet encourages using olive oil as the main fat. However, if you love butter and stick margarine as a spread, there are vegetable oil spreads available with lower saturated fat and zero trans fat.

What about Coconut Oil?

Coconut oil has made headlines as a miracle food, despite its high saturated fat content. The theory behind why coconut oil may have benefits is based on its medium-chain triglycerides, or MCTs. This type of fat is metabolized differently than the long-chain triglycerides (LCT) that make up the majority of liquid oils. One of the first popular claims was that coconut oil boosted weight loss because MCTs go directly from the intestine to the liver, so are less available to be stored as body fat. Even then, weight loss was a modest four pounds or so. Plus, this is based on custom-formulated 100 percent pure MCT oil vs. coconut oil, which is naturally about 40 to 60 percent MCT. As such, studies using coconut oil haven't shown meaningful weight loss.

When it comes to brain health, the theory is that a brain with dementia may have a harder time using glucose for energy (which means cells will starve), and that MCT in coconut oil provides an alternate fuel source to the brain in the form of ketones. However, the simple truth is that there is not nearly enough clinical data to back this up. Meanwhile, coconut oil is a substantial source of saturated fat that may do more harm than good.

Another claim is that coconut oil improves levels of HDL, or "good cholesterol." But all fats raise HDL somewhat. It's unsaturated fats from liquid oils like olive oil that will both lower LDL "bad cholesterol" and raise HDL. To point, a 2022 systematic review by Teng et al. concluded that coconut oil may be better for cholesterol levels than animal fats, but that it was not as healthful as other plant oils rich in polyunsaturated fats.

Nutrition science is an evolving field, but what we know today is that there isn't enough evidence to support that coconut oil is effective for the many ailments it claims to help, including Alzheimer's disease, heart disease, obesity, or diabetes. If you enjoy the taste of coconut oil, it can be kept in rotation in moderation, but based on what we know today, there are better options for brain health.

Cheese

The MIND diet recommends limiting whole-fat cheese to less than one serving a week, which means that if you enjoy cheese, to stick to having it once every couple weeks at most. The *Dietary Guidelines for Americans 2020–2025* and the American Heart Association recommend limiting it in a heart-healthy diet. The Dietary Guidelines recommend choosing fat-free or low-fat milk and yogurt instead of whole-fat cheese to reduce saturated fat and sodium intake while benefiting from vitamins A and D, and potassium in dairy foods.

Vegan cheeses offer a cholesterol-free option, though they may still be high in saturated fat. Take a look at the nutrition facts panel for more details and look for a saturated fat amount listed at below 10 percent of the Daily Value.

Pastries and Sweets

The MIND diet recommends limiting pastries and sweets to less than five times per week. The *Dietary Guidelines for Americans 2020–2025* discourages eating these foods not only because of their bad fats, but also because of their added sugar. These foods offer little to no positive nutrients. There is no need for these foods within a healthy diet, and they should only be included in very limited amounts.

Pastries and sweets include cookies, cakes, brownies, cupcakes, croissants, doughnuts, custards, ice cream, candy, and more. In addition to pastries and sweets, sugar-sweetened beverages such as soda, sports drinks, and any juice drink other than 100 percent juice should be limited.

Satisfy your sweet tooth naturally with whole fruit. They naturally contain sugars but in a reasonable ratio to its fiber, water, and total package of nutrition. In fact, berries such as blueberries and strawberries are sweet, nutritious, and an important component of the MIND diet.

Fried Fast Food

The MIND diet recommends limiting fried fast food to less than one serving per week. That means, at the most, having fried fast food once every two weeks, or about twice a month. The *Dietary Guidelines for Americans 2020–2025* recommends limiting fried foods because frying diminishes the healthfulness of any food. In fact, frying dilutes the nutrition in otherwise healthy foods such as poultry, fish, and vegetables, negating their brain health benefits.

If you find yourself at a fast food chain, you can still make smart choices. Look for the healthiest options on the menu. It may be a salad, with toppings and dressing on the side so you can choose whether and how much to consume. It may be a grilled chicken or grilled fish sandwich on whole wheat bread. Instead of French fries or chips, some chains offer healthier sides such as baby carrots. If you are served something with fried breading, you can choose to remove it before eating.

Many of the larger chains offer nutrition information on site and online and must produce it on request so you can make informed choices.

CHAPTER 5
THE NUTRIENTS

Understanding how key nutrients improve brain function helps improve the understanding of how the foods we see associated with better cognitive function may work, but there is still so much we don't know, which is why eating whole foods is your best bet. Nutrient-specific research provides an imperfect set of knowledge to begin with, and this chapter is not exhaustive. Instead, it is meant to provide an overview of some of the best-studied and most promising nutrients that are involved in cognitive aging, dementia, and cognitive development, from nutrients with antioxidant and anti-inflammatory action to those with a possible role in protecting against beta-amyloid deposits and cell death. This includes dietary fats, vitamin E, certain B vitamins (folate and B12), flavonoids, and carotenoids.

When thinking about individual nutrients distilled into supplements, it is important to understand the well-established nutrition principle that the intersection of nutrients and health fall on a U-shaped curve where getting too little leads to deficiency, and too much leads to toxicity. Good health is in between the extremes. Supplements can easily go overboard on nutrients, whereas food sources won't. That's why, with a few exceptions, taking a food-first approach is the ideal way for older adults to meet nutrient needs.

Good and Bad Fats

There is no max on total fat in the MIND diet, but the types and proportions of fats matter.

Good Fats

A 2021 meta-analysis found that omega-3 intake was associated with a reduced risk of mild cognitive impairment.[35] The PREDIMED trial tested a Mediterranean diet supplemented with healthy fats: either nuts or olive oil, and both were effective in producing higher cognitive scores compared to low-fat diets. Risk for Alzheimer's disease and cognitive decline goes down when unsaturated fats replace saturated and trans fats. The MIND diet emphasizes the use of olive oil as the main dietary fat, which is rich in monounsaturated fat as well as many polyphenols. Other sources of healthy fats include nuts, seeds, avocado, and seafood.

Bad Fats

Eating too much saturated and trans fats increases the risk of dementia. In a 2018 meta-analysis, Ruan et al. found that diets higher in saturated fat were associated with a higher risk of Alzheimer's disease and dementia. A 2020 study by Hill et al. found diets high in saturated fat are also associated with poorer cognition.

When it comes to unhealthy fats, animal studies show that diets high in saturated and trans fats lead to signs of dementia such as blood-brain barrier dysfunction, inflammation, and amyloid clusters. Several observational studies have also found that middle-age adults with high cholesterol are at an increased risk of developing dementia later in life.

---

35   Run-Ze Zhu et al., "Dietary Fatty Acids and Risk for Alzheimer's Disease, Dementia, and Mild Cognitive Impairment," *Nutrition* 90 (2021): 111355, https://doi.org/10.1016/j.nut.2021 .111355.

In one animal study, there was significant blood-brain barrier damage and inflammation after three months on a diet high in saturated fat. The functional damage was 30 times worse than at the start. The diet used in the study was 20 percent saturated fat, which equates to a little more than 44 grams of saturated fat for a 2,000-calorie diet. In another animal study, amyloid concentrations went up as a result of four months on a diet that was 40 percent saturated fat (nearly 90 grams of saturated fat for a 2,000 calorie diet). In a cell study, trans fat was found to favor the formation of sticky amyloid proteins seen in Alzheimer's disease while also discouraging a variation of the protein that does not result in amyloids. Studies also suggest that high-fat diets, especially when high in saturated fat, affect cognitive performance. Learning and memory skills declined in a long-term animal study of mice eating a diet that was 40 percent fat (versus 4.5 percent in the standard food). Based on nearly two decades of research in this area, the scientists concluded that a long-term high-fat diet disrupts the way the body uses glucose: the hippocampus region of the brain adapts to use less of it.

The easiest way to avoid saturated and trans fat is to avoid the brain-harming foods identified in the MIND diet. Another way to easily identify a saturated fat is to see if it is solid at room temperature.

Good vs. Bad Fats

In the research that adjusted for types of fat, results were consistent: the more saturated and trans fats there were in the diet, the higher the rates of cognitive decline. For example, replacing saturated fat with plant monounsaturated fats or linoleic acid was associated with lower rates of premature death from any cause, including Alzheimer's disease, according to a 2019 American Heart Association study. In addition, most of these studies found that higher intakes of monounsaturated (MUFA) and polyunsaturated (PUFA) fats did the reverse and led to a slowdown of cognitive decline. These findings are supported by lab studies in which animals eating diets higher in omega-3s (especially DHA, which is abundant in brain tissue), including older mice, did better at learning new things and remembering.

Why do some studies show mixed results? Some randomized trials using DHA omega-3 supplements didn't show any benefits for cognitive health. These trials allowed participants to eat fish up to three times per week, so the difference between treatment and placebo groups would have been nullified given that just one fish meal per week is adequate for reducing risk of dementia. There are also mixed results from several population studies of dietary fat and cognitive decline, but only when the methodology did not control for type of fat. Therefore, the mixed results are more likely due to poor research design and should be taken with a grain of salt, especially when the results from the majority of good-quality research is consistent.

Vitamin E

MIND diet foods that are naturally rich in vitamin E include olive oil, nuts, whole grains, and leafy green vegetables. Vitamin E is important to brain health. As an antioxidant nutrient, it protects the brain from the oxidative stress and damage to neural tissue that comes with being a site of high metabolic activity. A deficiency in this essential nutrient leads to a variety of brain-related symptoms, including cognitive decline, loss of control over the body's movement, lack of reflexes, paralyzed eye muscles, and decreased sensitivity to vibration, all of which decrease the ability to fully function in society.

Naturally occurring vitamin E comes in eight forms, but for our purposes we'll focus on the two most commonly studied ones, referred to by their chemical names: alpha-tocopherol and gamma-tocopherol. Both of these forms are found in food, and have antioxidant and anti-inflammatory properties. However, the vitamin E appearing on nutrition labels refers to alpha-tocopherol.

Several clinical trials using a vitamin E supplement found no benefit, and even some harm for cognitive decline and Alzheimer's disease. However, epidemiological studies, which are studies that observe and track health data for large populations over time, consistently show benefits of dietary (food-sourced) vitamin E for Alzheimer's prevention. Research has shown that higher levels of gamma-tocopherol in the brain is associated with less amyloid and neurofibrillary tangles. What's complicated is that some research shows that high levels of alpha-tocopherol (the main type found in supplements) but low gamma-tocopherol is associated with more amyloid build up. This could be why dietary sources are safe and helpful, but oversupplementation may be harmful.

In addition to being a strong antioxidant, vitamin E is involved in creating new brain cells (neurogenesis), helping them develop (neuronal differentiation), and supporting communication in the hippocampus where we hold short-term memories, transfer some into long-term storage, and process emotions (hippocampal synaptic functionality). A 2020 study found that higher levels of alpha- and gamma-tocopherol meant lower levels of activated microglia in some, but not all regions of the brain.[36] That's significant because activating microglia (the immune cells of the central nervous system) is associated with making neurofibrillary tangles worse and killing off neurons and synapses. This is supported by a 2021 study in centenarians that found that those with more vitamin E in their brains had fewer neurofibrillary tangles.[37]

The confusion around vitamin E's brain-health benefits is due to several studies on vitamin E supplements (in the form

---

36 F. A. de Leeuw et al., "Brain Tocopherol Levels Are Associated with Lower Activated Microglia Density in Elderly Human Cortex," *Alzheimers & Dementia* 6, no. 1 (2021): e12021.

37 J. Tanprasertsuk et al., "Brain A-Tocopherol Concentration Is Inversely Associated with Neurofibrillary Tangle Counts in Brain Regions Affected in Earlier Braak Stages: A Cross-Sectional Finding in the Oldest Old," *JAR Life* 10 (2021): 8–16.

of alpha-tocopherol), which showed no benefits for cognitive decline or Alzheimer's disease. These null results were supported by observational epidemiological studies (the kind of studies that follow large groups of people over several years) that looked at vitamin E supplementation and cognitive decline. These results were disappointing, especially after many animal studies had shown that alpha-tocopherol supported brain health. The few studies showing brain-protective effects of alpha-tocopherol supplementation were for people who started with low levels of vitamin E in their diet. Levels of vitamin E would need to be below 6.1 milligrams per day in order for supplements to have a positive effect, according to an analysis of nutrient insufficiency in older adult populations. Average intakes are about 7.2 mg per day, which is above this threshold, though still well below the recommended 15 mg per day.

The bottom line is that vitamin E from foods is preferable to vitamin E from supplements, which may do more harm than good, and at best, are still controversial. Good news: there is no controversy around vitamin E from foods, and both alpha-tocopherol and gamma-tocopherol from foods may reduce the rate of cognitive decline and Alzheimer's disease. The key difference is that the amounts found in foods are at much more moderate levels and work together to keep the brain healthy. Furthermore, foods may contain more of the eight vitamin E forms, not just the two that have been well studied. These other forms are also known to have antioxidant and anti-inflammatory properties. This is all the more reason to choose food first and to be cautious of reducing the benefits of whole foods to single nutrients. Natural sources of vitamin E include whole grains, nuts, and vegetable oils.

What else does vitamin E do for health? Vitamin E is an essential nutrient that the body cannot produce on its own (which is why it must come from the diet). It is an antioxidant, which means it protects the body against damage caused by free radicals. It helps keep the immune system strong, helps form red blood cells, helps the body use vitamin K, and assists in widening the blood vessels to keep blood from clotting inside them. Vitamin E is a fat-soluble vitamin, which means that the body needs dietary fat to absorb it and is why it's often found in naturally fatty foods like almonds.

Healthy eating patterns should include at least 20 percent of calories from fat. Any lower and it's hard to meet recommended intake levels of important fat-soluble nutrients such as vitamin E. The *Dietary Guidelines for Americans 2020–2025*, which de-emphasizes total fat limits and focuses more on the type of fat, recommends eating many foods that contain both healthy fats and vitamin E, such as vegetable oils, nuts, and seeds. Vitamin E is also commonly found in leafy green vegetables. Specific examples of natural food sources include olive oil, almonds, peanuts, sunflower seeds, beet greens, collard greens, spinach, and broccoli. The recommended daily value is 15 mg, with upper limits set at 1,000 mg per day for adults who are not pregnant or lactating. Eating vitamin E in foods is safe, but higher doses from supplements can increase the risk of bleeding in general, bleeding in the brain, and birth defects.

WHAT DOES VITAMIN E ON A LABEL MEAN?

Vitamin E on food or supplement labels only refers to alpha-tocopherols and should be listed in milligrams, according to the latest nutrition labelling policies. If you come across a label that still shows vitamin E in international units (IU), you may convert this to milligrams by multiplying by 0.67 for food sources, or by 0.45 for supplement sources. Synthetic vitamin E is less bioavailable, which is why the conversion factor is lower. In either case, it will be helpful to pay attention to the percent Daily Value listed on the nutrition facts panel. Foods that provide at least 10 percent of the Daily Value for vitamin E are considered a good source of that nutrient.

B Vitamins: Folate and B12

Folate (vitamin B9) and vitamin B12 (cobalamin) are both essential, water-soluble B vitamins that are often discussed together because they are involved in many of the same functions and are interrelated. Without enough of either, the body's red blood cell count goes down, reducing the ability to deliver oxygen to tissues. Vitamin B12 deficiency can result in cognitive impairment as well as fatigue, depression, anemia, and nerve damage that can cause tingling, numbness, burning, and loss of feeling in arms, hands, legs, and feet (also known as peripheral neuropathy). They are both involved in brain development early in life, as well as brain degeneration later in life.

These two vitamins are studied in relation to dementia because they help metabolize homocysteine, a substance that has been associated with an increased risk of developing Alzheimer's disease. Without enough folate and B12 in the diet, homocysteine accumulates in the body. B vitamin supplementation (folate, B12, and B6) was shown to be helpful in a study that targeted older adults with high homocysteine. Two years of treatment slowed down overall cognitive decline, including memory complaints.

However, the body of research on these two vitamins and dementia has been complicated by inconsistent findings. Ten population studies have looked at folate and B12 in relation to cognitive decline. Three showed protective effects for B12, and four had positive results for folate, but several had mixed results.

A paper by Dr. Martha Clare Morris, published in *Proceedings of the Nutrition Society*, describes methodology issues resulting in study designs that are not sensitive enough to show an effect. Some studies did not measure participants' starting levels for these nutrients, which is important because supplementation may only benefit people who have a need (that is, those with low B vitamin status). For example, among the several large, long-term trials, in the one that took starting folate levels into account, there was a benefit from folic acid supplementation in those with low folate status, resulting in a slower rate of cognitive decline. In a study that found no overall effect for B vitamin supplementation, there actually was a protective benefit when a later analysis of the data focused on participants who had low B vitamin levels at the start of the study.

Is It Possible to Get Too Much Folate?

Folic acid is the synthetic form of folate, and deficiency is now rare since the USDA mandated folic acid fortification of refined grains in 1998. They did so in response to the well-established role of folate in preventing fetal neural tube defects, and there's good evidence it helped dramatically reduce cases by 36 percent in its first 10 years (1996–2006). However, an unintended consequence is that older adults may be getting too much.

Folate, a water-soluble vitamin, isn't usually stored in the body; excesses are removed in the urine. However, some research shows that the liver doesn't easily metabolize folic acid (the form used in fortified foods and supplements) into the form of folate the body can use, resulting in high levels of unmetabolized folic acid circulating in the blood. A study among CHAP participants found that people with folic acid intakes above the recommended daily 400 micrograms experienced faster cognitive decline. Similar results were reported in a study of the large National Health and Nutrition Examination Survey (NHANES) data, in which low B12 and high folate led to impaired cognitive performance compared to people with normal levels of folate.

Is it possible to get too much vitamin B12 from supplements? Vitamin B12 from food isn't well-absorbed by up to 30 percent of older adults as the stomach become less acidic with aging, but because B12 can be stored in the liver for three to five years, deficiency and its related cognitive damage could be developing years before signs of anemia reveal it. In this case, supplements may be a good choice.

In summary, the current evidence suggests that being folate or vitamin B12 deficient speeds up cognitive decline, and low folate may also increase the risk of Alzheimer's disease (no such relationship has been established for B12). Excessive folate may also speed up cognitive decline, especially if B12 is low. Folate naturally found in foods isn't likely to add up to high levels, but vitamin supplements and foods made with fortified grains can contribute to high folic acid intake.

Overall, fixing low intakes of B vitamins may help with cognitive decline, but people who are already getting enough folate and B12 won't necessarily benefit more from adding more. Future randomized clinical trials should target people with low intakes to truly test if there's a solid cause and effect.

In the meantime, natural food sources of folate, but supplement or fortified food sources of B12, are ideal. Foods that naturally provide folate include dark green vegetables like broccoli, spinach, brussels sprouts, artichokes, and collard greens, and legumes such as edamame, chickpeas, lentils, beans, and peas. Vitamin B12 is only found naturally in animal foods such as fish and poultry, but is in some fortified milk alternatives (e.g., soy milk, rice milk, almond milk), soy-based meat alternatives, and other fortified foods.

DID YOU KNOW?

Folate is also known as vitamin B9 but became commonly known as folate—a term related to the Latin word for leaf (folium)—in the 1940s when it was established that B9 could be found in leafy green vegetables such as spinach, collard greens, butter lettuce, and bok choy. Today, we know that in addition to leafy greens, legumes are also a consistent source of folate, especially lentils, beans, and peas.

Flavonoids and Carotenoids

The brain is a busy place, and all that metabolic activity puts it at risk for oxidative stress and tissue damage. Antioxidant enzymes in the body are not as available to the brain as antioxidant nutrients from food, making them especially important to the aging brain. The antioxidant vitamin E was discussed at length earlier, but there are two additional classes of antioxidants that may help: carotenoids and flavonoids. The MIND diet provides plenty of both, especially from leafy greens and berries.

Flavonoids are biologically active polyphenolic compounds important to good health that occur naturally in a wide range of plant foods, including fruit, vegetables, chocolate, nuts, wine, and tea. There are six major subclasses of flavonoids: anthocyanidins, flavan-3-ols, flavonols, flavanols, flavanones, and isoflavones. They are studied for health benefits related to cardiovascular disease, glycemic control and diabetes, certain cancers, and cognitive function. Major sources of flavonoids include berries such as blueberries, strawberries, raspberries, elderberries, and European black currants; vegetables such as eggplant, red peppers, and purple cabbage; beans such as chickpeas; whole grains like quinoa; and other foods such as black, green, and oolong tea, oranges, grapefruit, lemons, onions, bananas, tomatoes, parsley, mint, rosemary, and oregano.

Carotenoids are naturally occurring yellow/green, orange, and red pigments made by plants, many of which have antioxidant properties. The most common carotenoids in the American diet are alpha-carotene, beta-carotene, lycopene, lutein, zeaxanthin, and beta-cryptoxanthin. Eating carotenoid foods is linked to a reduced risk of cardiovascular disease, some cancers, age-related macular degeneration, and cataracts. Carotenoids are best absorbed when eaten with fat, such as olive oil.

Top sources of carotenoids include:
- Leafy greens such as spinach, kale, and collard greens
- Vegetables such as carrots, sweet potato, butternut squash, red bell pepper, tomatoes (technically a fruit), pumpkin, brussels sprouts, and broccoli
- Fruits such as apricots, persimmon, cantaloupe, oranges, watermelon, and tomatoes
- Other foods such as eggs, paprika, chili peppers, shrimp, crab, and salmon

There are no specific recommendations for flavonoids or carotenoids established by the US government (other than the carotenoids that contribute to total vitamin A intake), so the best way to ensure adequate intake is to eat a variety of plant foods, including various vegetables, nuts, whole grains, beans, fruit, seafood, and even foods like spices and eggs.

PART TWO

Your MIND Diet Plan

The MIND diet does nobody any good unless it is put into practice. This section of the book helps you create your own MIND diet plan. As a reminder, the MIND diet has 15 components: 10 types of food to eat and five to limit, for a total possible weekly score of 15. Points are awarded for eating more brain-healthy foods and successfully limiting the brain-harming foods. While a perfect score of 15 is admirable, you don't need to attain perfection to benefit from the MIND diet. So do what you can today and add on from there when you're ready. Remember that the most therapeutic MIND diet scores seen in the original research ranged from 8.5 to 12.5.

CHAPTER 6
WHAT TO EAT (AND LIMIT)

For reference, the top-scoring participants in the MIND studies ate about 1,800 calories per day, but your individual needs may be higher or lower depending on physical activity and weight management goals. In general, the "what to eat" list is a starting point and you are welcome and encouraged to eat more of these healthy foods—with the exception of wine. Conversely, consider the "what to limit" list a set of maximums that you strive to stay well below. It's best to work with a registered dietitian to meet your individual needs. Below are the MIND guidelines to get you started.

THE EAT LIST

Serving sizes	• Vegetables: 1 cup fresh leafy greens, ½ cup cooked leafy greens, ½ cup other vegetables • Whole grains: ½ cup cooked • Nuts: 1 ounce (about ¼ cup) • Beans: ½ cup cooked • Berries: ½ cup fresh, ¼ cup dried • Poultry: 3 ounces cooked (about 4 to 5 ounces raw) • Fish: 3 ounces cooked (about 4 to 5 ounces raw) • Olive oil: 1 tablespoon • Wine: 5 ounces
Daily	• 3 servings of whole grains • 1 serving of vegetables (non-leafy greens) • 1 glass of wine • Olive oil
6 days a week	• 1 serving of leafy greens
5 days a week	• 1 serving of nuts
Every other day (4 days/week)	• 1 serving of beans
Twice a week	• 1 serving of berries • 1 serving of poultry (not fried)
Once a week	• 1 serving of fish (not fried)

Limit foods on the following list as much as possible. This is about limiting, but not necessarily eliminating any foods. If zero tolerance is not practical, aim to limit these foods according to the below guidelines.

THE LIMIT LIST

Serving sizes	• Butter or margarine: 1 tablespoon
	• Pastries and sweets: 1 to 5 ounces (check the label), below are some examples:
	  –Cookies: 2 pieces (1 ounce)
	  –Light/medium cakes (e.g., coffee cake, doughnuts, angel food cake): 1 medium doughnut (2 to 3 ounces)
	  –Heavy cakes (e.g., cheesecake, pie): 1 slice (4 to 5 ounces)
	• Ice cream: ½ cup
	• Red meat: 3 ounces cooked (about 4 to 5 ounces raw)
	• Whole-fat cheese: 1 ounce
	• Fried fast food: Any (e.g., 1 medium order of French fries)

Avoid daily	• 1 serving of butter or margarine
Avoid most days (5 days/week)	• 1 serving of pastries or sweets
Avoid most days (4 days/week)	• 1 serving of red meat
Avoid weekly (1 day/week)	For cheese and fried fast food, the recommendation is to limit to less than once a week, so if they are consumed one week, the next week would have to eliminate them completely. • 1 serving of fried fast food • 1 serving of whole-fat cheese

Keeping Score

Before even getting started with the MIND diet, it would be interesting to score your current diet for a week based on the MIND model. This will provide a baseline, and you can track progress from this point. This may be enough to help you make changes in the right direction. Start tracking your diet using the MIND Diet Weekly Scoreboard, and if you'd like more detailed help, go on to the menu-planning worksheets.

A simple way to track your weekly progress is to make check marks for every serving of MIND foods—from all 15 groups—that you've eaten/avoided each meal. At the end of the week, tally your score and see how you fared. Remember that in the MIND studies, those who scored in the top two tiers were not perfect and still benefited. Tier one scored 12.5 to 8.5 and tier two scored 7 to 8 points, and both were linked to a reduced risk of Alzheimer's disease.

MIND Diet Weekly Scorecard

Use a blank meal planning grid to fill in your meals for the week and tally up your score accordingly. See the next page for example templates.

Sample
MIND DIET WEEKLY MEAL PLAN

	Sun	Mon	Tue	
Breakfast				
Lunch				
Snack				
Dinner				
Snack				

Sample
MIND DIET WEEKLY MEAL PLAN

	Wed	Thu	Fri	Sat

Sample
MIND DIET WEEKLY SCORECARD

	Sun	Mon	Tue	Wed	
Leafy greens 6 times (6+ cups)/week					
More vegetables 7 times (7+ Half cups)/week					
Nuts 5 times (5+ oz)/week)					
Beans 4 times (4+ Half cups)/week					
Berries 2 times (2+ Half cups)/week					
Lean poultry 2 times (2+ servings, 3 oz)/week					
Seafood 1 time (1+ serving, 3 oz)/week					
Olive oil Main fat daily					
Whole grains 21 times (21+ Half cups)/week					
Wine 7 glasses (5 oz)/day—optional					
Butter Less than 7 Tbsp/week					
Red meat Less than 4 (3 oz) servings/week					
Pastries & sweets Less than 5 servings/week					
Cheese Less than 1 oz/week					
Fried fast foods Less than once/week					

Sample
MIND DIET WEEKLY SCORECORD

	Thurs	Fri	Sat	TOTAL	SCORE
			Total Mind Score:	

Simple Scoring

Give yourself a "1" for each MIND diet target you achieved. For example, if you had fish once during the week, you'd have a score of "1" for that food group because you met the target. If you had berries three times (target: twice a week), you'd have a score of "1" for that food group too, even though you exceeded the goal. If you missed the target goal, you'd give yourself a "0."

MIND TARGET SERVINGS PER WEEK

SERVINGS OF FOODS TO EAT	SERVING SIZE	
Whole grains (per day)	½ cup cooked	
Vegetables (per week), applies to non-leafy green vegetables	½ cup cooked	
Leafy greens (per week)	1 cup fresh or ½ cup cooked	
Nuts (per week)	¼ cup (1 ounce)	
Beans (per week)	½ cup cooked	
Berries (per week)	½ cup	
Poultry (per week)	3 ounces cooked	
Fish (per week)	3 ounces cooked or 4 ounces raw	
Wine (as noted)	5 ounces	
Olive oil (per day)	Used as primary oil	
SERVINGS OF FOODS TO AVOID	SERVING SIZE	
Butter (per day)	1 tablespoon	
Pastries, sweets (per week)	1 to 5 ounces (check the label), see examples above.	
Red meat (per week)	3 ounces cooked	
Whole-fat cheese (per week)	1 ounce	
Fried fast food (per week)	1 regular order	

Advanced Scoring

For a more accurate, but slightly more complicated assessment, you can give yourself partial points for reaching partial goals. A scoring guideline follows.

SCORES		
0	**0.5**	**1**
< 1	1-2	3+
0-4	5-6	7+
0-2	3-5	6+
< ¼ serving	¼-4	5+
0	1-3	4+
0	1	2+
0	1	2+
0	¼-¾	1+
Never or > 1/day	1 glass a month–6 times per week	1
Not used	n/a	Primary oil used
0	**0.5**	**1**
> 2	1-2	< 1
7+	5-6	0-4
7+	4-6	0-3
7+	1-6	< 1
4+	1-3	<1

CHAPTER 7

MEAL PLANNING

Meal planning is essential to implementing your MIND diet plan. With a little forethought and some helpful meal-planning tools, successfully following the MIND diet can be simple and efficient. The good news is that unlike other diets that ask you to translate grams of nutrients into food, the MIND diet is already based on real food. The researchers have laid the scientific foundation. All you have to worry about is deciding what goes on your plate, and the nutrient levels will take care of themselves.

The worksheets that follow will help organize food lists and menu ideas for the week. There are sample worksheets already filled out with examples, followed by blank templates for you to put your MIND diet into action.

Planning Your Food Choices

The below worksheet is filled out with food choices in each food group. It shows a range of options to give you some ideas. However, in real life, it is more practical to stick to some of the same foods for multiple meals. For example, if you roast a pan of brussels sprouts for dinner one night and have leftovers, they can be one of the vegetable servings for the following day. Or, if you make a large batch of brown rice, it could be used for a serving at lunch and two more servings at dinner to meet the daily recommended three servings.

When you fill out your own worksheet, the result should be a list of foods that fit the MIND diet guidelines as well as your personal preferences. It's also helpful because knowing what's in your mental "cupboard" of options is a natural way to start menu planning with a concrete set of options in hand. This step makes the menu planning stage much less daunting.

Serving sizes

- **Vegetables:** 1 cup fresh leafy greens, ½ cup cooked leafy greens, ½ cup other vegetables
- **Whole grains:** ½ cup cooked
- **Nuts:** 1 ounce (about ¼ cup)
- **Beans:** ½ cup cooked
- **Berries:** ½ cup fresh, ¼ cup dried
- **Poultry:** 3 ounces cooked (about 4 to 5 ounces raw)
- **Fish:** 3 ounces cooked (about 4 to 5 ounces raw)
- **Olive oil:** 1 tablespoon
- **Wine:** 5 ounces
- **Butter or margarine:** 1 tablespoon
- **Pastries and sweets:** 1 to 5 ounces
- **Red meat:** 3 ounces cooked (about 4 to 5 ounces raw)
- **Whole-fat cheese:** 1 ounce
- **Fried fast food:** 1 regular order (e.g., medium order of French fries)

Sample
MIND FOODS WORKSHEET

	Sun	Mon	Tue
Whole grains (WG) 3/day	Brown rice Barley Oats Fonio	Buckwheat Corn Farro	Bulgur Freekeh Einkorn
Vegetables (non-leafy greens) 1/day	Broccoli Butternut squash Tomatoes	Carrots Cauliflower Fennel	Sweet potatoes Asparagus Radishes
Leafy greens 6+/week	Kale Butter lettuce	Spinach Spring mix Microgreens	Arugula Watercress
Nuts 5+/week	-	Walnuts	Almonds
Beans 4+/week	Black beans	-	Pinto beans
Berries 2+/week	-	-	Blueberries
Poultry 2+/week	Skinless chicken breast	-	-
Fish 1+/week	-	-	Wild salmon
Olive oil use as primary oil	2 T	2 T	2 T
Wine 1/day	5 oz Cabernet franc wine	5 oz Cabernet sauvignon wine	5 oz Pinot Noir wine

Sample
MIND FOODS WORKSHEET

Wed	Thu	Fri	Sat
Millet White quinoa Rye	Popcorn Spelt Sorghum	Whole wheat pasta Teff Wild rice	Triticale Red rice Black or red quinoa
Brussels sprouts Bok choy	Green beans Snow peas	Beets Sugar snap peas Bell peppers	Zucchini Eggplant Mushrooms
Cabbage Endive	Collard greens Beet greens	Romaine lettuce Swiss chard	-
Pepitas	Pecans	Peanuts	-
-	Kidney beans	-	Chickpeas
-	-	Strawberries	-
Lean ground turkey	-	-	-
-	-	-	-
2 T	2 T	2 T	2T
5 oz Temperanillo wine	5 oz Rosé wine	5 oz Merlot wine	5 oz Malbec wine

Sample
MIND FOODS WORKSHEET

	Sun	Mon	Tue	
Whole-fat cheese* <1/week Max: 0-1/week	1 oz cheddar cheese	-	-	
Fried fast food* <1/week Max: 0-1/week	-	1 small order of French fries	-	
Red meat* <4/week Max: 3/week	-	-	3 oz steak	
Pastries or sweets* <5/week Max: 4/week	2 small cookies	1 small blueberry muffin	-	
Butter or margarine* <1T/d Max: 6.99 T/week	1 tsp butter	1 tsp butter	1 tsp butter	

*Limit these foods as much as possible. Examples of prudent maximum amounts of these foods are listed purely for illustration. It is better if you can avoid them altogether. For cheese and fast food, the recommendation is to limit to less than once a week, so if the below foods were consumed one week, the next week would have to eliminate them completely.

Sample
MIND FOODS WORKSHEET

Wed	Thu	Fri	Sat
-	-	-	
-	-	-	
-	1 small hamburger	-	3 oz meatballs
-	1 small croissant	-	1 small brownie
1 tsp butter	1 tsp margarine	1 tsp margarine	1 tsp margarine

Sample MIND Menu Worksheet

Below is what a week on the MIND diet could look like. Full of healthy, whole foods, it's not just brain food, it's heart-healthy and diabetes-friendly, and provides lasting energy that will fill you up but won't slow you down thanks to the filling fiber and balance of healthy proteins and fats. Use the blank MIND Menu Worksheet following to fill in your own menu ideas.

Sample
MIND DIET WEEKLY MEAL PLAN

	Sun	Mon	Tue	
Breakfast	Mini frittatas & whole grain toast	Drink your greens smoothie	Berry fonio	
Lunch	Farro salad with chopped herbed chicken	Farro salad with chopped herbed chicken	Cauliflower soup with whole wheat baguette toast points	
Snack	No-bake chewy granola balls	No-bake chewy granola balls	Ginger-citrus vitality bites	
Dinner	Garden pie with Purple is the new pink mocktail	Chana masala with brown basmati rice and side of greens, with glass of wine	Turkey chili with whole wheat bread roll, crisp greens & grapes salad, and glass of wine	
Snack	Greek yogurt with port wine reduction and walnuts	Creamy no-cook PB&J mousse	Mini choco-peanut cup	

Sample
MIND DIET WEEKLY MEAL PLAN

Wed	Thu	Fri	Sat
Smoked trout toast	PB&J steel cut oats	Maca mocha smoothie	Open-faced omelet with smoked trout, whole grain toast, and turmeric wellness shot
Power greens with chicken and sherry vinaigrette	Turkey chili with whole wheat bread roll	Beets & berries barley salad with poached chicken	Bibim guksu buckwheat noodle bowl
Crunchy spiced chickpeas	Blueberry cinnamon smoothie	Berry parfait	Ruby red veggie veggie dip with crudite
Pan-seared salmon with warm fonio and asparagus pilaf with warm grapes, with glass of wine	Tipsy prunes & pork with shaved brussels sprouts, figs, & fennel salad, plus a wine	Fish tacos with glass of wine	Chicken shawarma pita pockets with glass of wine
No-bake chewy granola balls	Walnut-stuffed apricots	Almond-citrus chocolate bites	Mini choco-peanut cup

Creating Your Own Meal Plans: Blank Worksheet

See page 132 for a weekly meal-planning template.

Food Safety

Cooking is an act of caring and generosity. You want your dishes to be delicious and nourishing, but first and foremost you want to ensure that they won't make anyone sick from food safety mistakes.

Food safety—from shopping to preparation and storage—is important for everyone, but especially the very young, older adults, anyone with a compromised immune system, and anyone responsible for providing food to these groups. The risk of food poisoning is higher in these groups, and the consequences can be severe.

For these groups, it is recommended to only eat seafood, meat, poultry, or eggs that have been fully cooked to safe temperatures; avoid sprouts, raw juice, raw milk, and anything made from unpasteurized milk (e.g., this category could include Brie, Camembert, Asadero, Panela, queso blanco, queso fresco, yogurt, pudding, ice cream, and frozen yogurt, if made from unpasteurized milk—check the label); and heat up deli meats to kill listeria bacteria.

Below are general guidelines that anyone working with food should embrace.

1. **Wash hands well, and wash them often.** That means washing hands with soap for at least 20 seconds. When working with food, wash hands, at a minimum, before starting to cook, after handling raw meat, and after food prep is finished. While washing up after raw meat is a must, it doesn't hurt to wash in between preparing other foods too (e.g., between

chopping an onion and chopping greens), as bacteria can cross-contaminate between any foods.

2. **Separate foods that could cross-contaminate each other.** That means having separate cutting boards for raw meat versus fruits and vegetables, and using different knives to work with each. If that's not possible, be sure to thoroughly wash and sanitize knives before switching foods. Also, fruits and vegetables should be rinsed before coming to the cutting board to reduce the risk of transferring bacteria to the cutting board. All cutting boards and knives should be washed well with hot water and soap after use. Old cutting boards with visible grooves (where bacteria can hide) should be replaced. Wipe down and sanitize counters and cooking areas before and after food prep.

3. **Be aware of food temperatures.** Keep hot foods hot (above 140°F), cold foods cold (below 40°F), and frozen foods freezing (below 0°F). Bacteria love to grow between 40°F –140°F, and will multiply in the right conditions. Don't leave prepared food out for more than two hours. On hotter days, cut that time down to no more than an hour. Make sure your refrigerator is maintaining a temperature of 40°F or below.

4. **Be aware of cooking temperatures.** Raw meat, fish, and poultry must be cooked to safe temperatures. Poultry must be cooked to 165°F. Fresh seafood must be cooked to 145°F (for shellfish, cook until the flesh is opaque; for clams, mussels, and oysters, cook until their shells open). Red meat needs to be cooked to 145°F, unless it is ground, which needs to reach 160°F. Food thermometers are an essential kitchen tool to confirm internal cooking temperatures.

5. **There's a right way to refrigerate hot food.** Store hot food in small, shallow containers, which provide more surface area to allow the food to cool down quickly and evenly, so

bacteria has less chance to find a comfortable environment to grow in. The down side is that introducing hot food into the refrigerator makes the refrigerator work harder. To minimize this effect, place all the hot foods in storage containers before opening the refrigerator door, then place at the bottom back of the refrigerator (the coldest area), before quickly closing the door again. You may also choose to quick-chill hot foods by surrounding them with ice packs for 20 minutes before transferring to the refrigerator.

6. **Defrost food in the refrigerator or the microwave.** Gone are the days when it is considered safe to defrost food on the kitchen counter.

7. **Don't overstuff the refrigerator.** Some space is required for cool air to flow and do its job. Taking stock of the refrigerator's contents is good policy anyway. It ensures you are regularly eating your perishable foods and that you don't keep past-due food lurking at the back of your refrigerator. At least once a week, check your refrigerator for any foods that need to be discarded.

8. **Keep your sink, counters, refrigerator drawers, utensil drawers, buttons, and handles, contamination-free.** Wash all these areas regularly with soap and water, and replace or sanitize kitchen sponges often, at least weekly. Soaked sponges can be microwaved for a minute or two, or run in the dishwasher with the dry heat setting, to help sanitize them. Scrub sponges can be saturated with a quarter cup of water and microwaved for a minute; cellulose sponges can be soaked in a Half cup of water and microwaved for two minutes.

9. **Wash all fruits and vegetables except those that are labeled as prewashed and ready to eat.**

10. **Do not rinse raw seafood, meat, and poultry.** It turns out that rinsing can do more harm, spreading bacteria rather than washing it away.

Food Safety: Leafy Greens

Below are additional tips specifically for green, leafy vegetables, which are often eaten raw. Raw foods raise inherent food safety concerns. Leafy greens are very healthy foods, so it's worth the effort to learn the simple techniques to ensure they're safe to eat. To keep leafy greens safe, it's all about prevention and avoiding the introduction of bad bacteria—from the farm all the way up until it reaches the fork.

1. **Buy from growers or brands you trust.** From the farm to the grocery store, your power is in choosing from trusted producers and retailers.

2. **Starting at the grocery store, be sure greens are in a refrigerated area.** Don't buy anything that looks wilted or brown. While shopping and when checking out, keep greens bagged and separated from raw meat and poultry.

3. **Once at home, store fresh leafy greens in a clean refrigerator at 40°F or below.** Continue to keep leafy greens and raw meat stored separately.

4. **Before and after handling fresh leafy greens, wash hands for 20 seconds with warm water and soap.** Outer leaves of greens can be thrown out. Cut away any parts that look damaged or bruised.

5. **Wash leafy greens thoroughly, which can help reduce bacteria that may be present.** Rinse all the greens, even the small, tightly packed leaves at the center of a head of lettuce. Soak greens in cool water, agitate them gently, let any debris sink, then lift them out of the bowl into a colander (this is important since draining alone simply adds the debris back

into the mix), and rinse under running water. The agitate-and-soak process can be repeated two to three times for crinkly greens (anything that's not totally flat-leafed), such as spinach, before rinsing.

6. **Packaged greens can look alike, prewashed or not.** If you want the convenience of pre-washed greens, look for the terms "prewashed," "triple-washed," or "ready to eat." Prewashed greens don't technically need another wash at home (and are washed in facilities that are cleaner than the average home kitchen).

7. **Cooking for 15 seconds at 160°F is all it takes to kill bacteria that may be on your greens.** The leafy greens that work well when cooked are hardier greens such as kale, collards, bok choy, and spinach.

8. **Organic greens should be washed with just as much care as conventionally grown greens.**

Stocking Your Kitchen

A well-stocked pantry is the foundation to any meal. Keep healthy staples on hand, and a nourishing meal will always be in reach. For items in cans or boxes, look for BPA-free cans or aseptic packaging.

Dry Pantry

- **Vegetables:** Corn, garlic, onions, potatoes, tomatoes (whole, diced, crushed, pureed, or made into a paste), roasted red peppers
- **Beans:** Black, cannellini, chickpeas, great northern, navy, pinto, red kidney
- **Fish:** Trout, tuna, anchovy fillets or paste

- **Whole grains:** Barley, brown rice, bulgur, farro, fonio, pasta (whole grain, assorted shapes), popping corn, quinoa, steel-cut oats, wild rice
- **Oil:** Extra-virgin olive oil, grapeseed oil, flaxseed oil, perilla seed oil
- **Wine:** Red (cabernet sauvignon, pinot noir), white (chardonnay, sauvignon blanc)
- **Other:** Herbs and spices (chili powder, crushed red pepper, curry powder, cinnamon, cumin, garlic powder, ginger, oregano, paprika, black pepper, rosemary, salt, thyme, turmeric)
- **Other:** Vinegars (distilled, apple cider, red wine, rice wine, champagne, balsamic)
- **Other:** Capers or olives, lentils, low-sodium vegetable broth, low-sodium chicken broth, coffee, tea

Freezer

- **Vegetables:** Broccoli, carrots, edamame, green beans, peas
- **Leafy greens:** Kale, spinach
- **Nuts:** Walnuts, almonds, peanuts, pecans, cashews
- **Berries:** Blueberries, raspberries, strawberries
- **Poultry:** Boneless, skinless chicken breasts, ground turkey
- **Fish:** Salmon, shrimp
- **Whole grains:** Cooked rice, bread
- **Other:** Sesame seeds, perilla seeds, hemp seeds, chia seeds, flaxseeds

Refrigerator

- **Vegetables:** Bell peppers, broccoli, carrots, cauliflower, celery, garlic, ginger root, onions, tomatoes, brussels sprouts, cauliflower, bok choy, winter squash, summer squash, mushrooms

- **Leafy greens:** Arugula, chard, kale, spinach, spring mix, romaine
- **Nuts:** Walnuts, almonds, peanuts, pecans, cashews
- **Other:** Sesame seeds, perilla seeds, hemp seeds, chia seeds, flaxseeds
- **Other:** Hot sauce, lemons, mustard (Dijon, whole grain), soy sauce

CHAPTER 8
RECIPES

The MIND diet is simpler than many "diets." There are no calories to count or long lists of foods to avoid. The eating pattern is based on food, not specific nutrients or overly prescriptive diet rules. This is about everyday eating. Simply follow the basic guidelines of the MIND diet—eat from the 10 basic brain-healthy food groups, limit the five brain-harming ones—and rest assured that you're doing something good for your brain health and overall well-being.

This chapter features over 60 recipes. Expect a range of options from simple smoothies to port wine reductions, traditional flavor combinations to internet-famous pairings, quick sides, never-boring salads, and so much more. I pull from my experiences as an American, Korean, world traveler, and netizen (citizen of the internet). Each recipe has nutrition information per serving and lists which MIND foods are included, so it's easy to see what foods are accounted for.

You'll notice there are no categories for breakfast, lunch, or dinner, and that is because you have the freedom to choose from any of the categories to make your meals. Have breakfast for dinner if you want; you're in charge.

I hope you enjoy these recipes and that you'll let me know if you try them.

Before You Get Started

A few important notes before you dig in:

- Use Diamond Crystal kosher salt or substitute with half the amount of salt called for if using table salt or Morton's kosher salt. All recipes were developed and tested with Diamond Crystal kosher salt, which is what is used in most professional settings. Good news, it's widely available. It also has less sodium for the same volume of salt (e.g., per ¼ teaspoon). Thanks to the patented way Diamond Crystal kosher salt is formed into hollow crystals, it offers more control and reduces the chances of overseasoning a dish.

- Stovetop recipes were tested on an induction stovetop, which emits fewer emissions into the home environment. They also cook about 5 to 10 percent faster than gas or electric stoves. Add a little more time to each step when using these types of stovetops. Keep in mind that even the same type of stoves may cook differently anyway, so it's best to look for doneness cues and let your taste (and other senses) be your ultimate guide.

- Special equipment that's helpful for recipes is noted, but we will assume you have: colanders, wire mesh strainers, cutting boards, knives, peelers, a blender, measuring cups and spoons, can opener, mixing bowls, pots and pans with lids, sheet pans, wire racks, baking dishes, spatulas, kitchen tongs, kitchen spoons, kitchen shears, whisks, serving ware, various sizes of plates, bowls, and glasses.

Culinary tips:

- Use a mixing bowl (or any large bowl) as a discard bowl to toss odds and ends into as you go. It will make clean-up simpler.
- Be aware that some spices (e.g., turmeric) can stain clothes and counters, etc. That's because they are concentrated sources of antioxidants, which impart color. Use glass and stainless steel

containers (which won't stain), wash hands often, and be aware of what comes into contact with the spices. Another pro tip: use chopsticks to pick up finger foods that may stain (like the Ginger-Citrus Vitality Bites on page 172).

- Liquid measurements should be taken at eye level unless you have a top-down measuring cup specially designed to measure liquids from above.
- When measuring flour, stir to fluff, lightly spoon it into a measuring cup or spoon, then level it with something flat, like a butter knife, spatula, chopstick, handle of another measuring spoon, etc.
- Brown sugar, date paste, and prune puree should be measured tightly packed.
- Sticky liquids are, well, sticky. Spray measuring cups with cooking spray or use oil and a paper towel to create a light barrier layer; then measure honey, maple syrup, etc. That way, it will more easily transfer out of the measuring cup and you will have the correct amount intended for your recipe.

Maggie's favorite kitchen tools

- Citrus zester
- Microplane (mesh safety gloves available)
- Vitamix blender
- Nutribullet personal inverted blender
- Thermoworks instant-read thermometer
- Silicone baking mats
- Silicone muffin pans
- Top-down measuring cups
- Mercer's Rules food ruler
- Kitchen scale
- Electric water kettle
- Large ice cube silicone trays
- Duralex prep bowls
- Pyrex mixing bowls
- Kitchen-Aid mini food chopper
- Cuisinart food processor
- Immersion blender
- OXO mini citrus juicer
- Glasslock glass food storage containers
- Enamel-coated cast-iron Dutch oven

HELPFUL CONVERSIONS

3 teaspoons	1 tablespoon
4 tablespoons	¼ cup
5 tablespoon + 1 teaspoon	⅓ cup
8 tablespoons	½ cup
16 tablespoons	1 cup
1 medium lemon	2 to 3 tablespoons juice (varies by lemon) 2 tablespoons loosely packed zest
1 medium lime	2 tablespoons (varies by lime) 2 teaspoons loosely packed zest
1 (15-ounce) can of beans	1½ cups beans
4 ounces raw fish, pork, or poultry	3 ounces cooked
1 tablespoon white sugar	1 tablespoon date paste
1 tablespoon honey or maple syrup	2 tablespoons date paste
2 teaspoons parmesan cheese	1 teaspoon nutritional yeast

Smoothies

DRINK YOUR GREENS SMOOTHIE

This one is for anyone who gets tired of salad. There's nothing wrong with drinking your greens every once in a while. Baby spinach is milder than its grown-up version, so it's less bitter. Parsley and lemon add vegetal and bright notes, and the sweet pineapple and punchy ginger make you forget you're drinking your greens. This smoothie is an excellent source of protein, vitamin B6, and folate and a good source of fiber, calcium, iron, potassium, and vitamin B12.

MIND foods: Leafy greens, beans
Yield: 1 serving | **Time:** 5 minutes

1 cup packed baby spinach
¼ cup packed flat-leaf parsley
juice from half a lemon
½ cup cold unsweetened soy milk

¼ cup regular low-fat plain yogurt
1 cup frozen pineapple chunks
2 teaspoons chopped peeled fresh
  ginger

1. Add the ingredients to a blender in the order listed. Blend on high for 30–60 seconds, until smooth. Transfer to a 20-ounce glass. Enjoy immediately.

Notes: Use a spoon with a thin edge and gentle pressure to scrape off the ginger peel. Any blender will work, but lower-powered blenders may require a longer blend time. If pineapple chunks are frozen into a block, run the closed package under hot water to loosen pieces, then pound with a heavy meat tenderizer or pot to break the pieces apart. Use the fruit as soon as possible, as freezing into a block is a sign of poor storage or freezer burn.

Substitution options: Try prewashed baby spinach for easy prep. For a thicker smoothie, start with ¼ cup soy milk, adding more until preferred consistency is reached. To make it less gingery, use 1 teaspoon instead of 2. To make it less tart, omit the lemon juice. To make this vegan, use soft silken tofu instead of yogurt.

Nutrition: 200 calories, 290 mg omega-3s, 1 g saturated fat, 12 g protein, 32 g carbohydrates, 4 g fiber, 0 g added sugars, 850 mg potassium, 0.4 mg vitamin B6, 150 mcg folate, 0.3 mcg vitamin B12, 40 mg choline, 4500 mcg lutein

STRAWBERRY LEMONADE SMOOTHIE

Strawberry lemonade is a fan favorite, especially when temperatures start to rise. Unlike regular strawberry lemonade, this smoothie offers fiber and protein, but no added sugar. This smoothie is rich in fiber, potassium, vitamin B6, and folate and a good source of protein and iron.

MIND foods: Berries, beans

Yield: 1 serving | **Time:** 5 minutes

½ cup cold unsweetened soy milk
zest from 1 lemon
juice from ½ lemon

1 medium frozen ripe banana, broken into 3–4 pieces
1 cup frozen strawberries

1. Add the ingredients to a blender in the order listed and blend on high for 30–60 seconds, until smooth. Transfer to a 10- to 12-ounce glass. Enjoy immediately.

Notes: It's important to use ripe bananas. Under-ripe bananas will be too bitter. Let bananas ripen and soften. Peels should be spotted. Then peel and break bananas into 3–4 pieces each and store in the freezer in a freezer-safe container. I do this in batches of 5–7 bananas at a time so I always have frozen banana pieces ready for smoothies.

> **Nutrition:** 250 calories, 300 mg omega-3s, 1 g saturated fat, 8 g protein, 50 g carbohydrates, 9 g fiber, 0 g added sugars, 1000 mg potassium, 0.6 mg vitamin B6, 100 mcg folate, 0 mcg vitamin B12, 30 mg choline, 90 mcg lutein

BLUEBERRY CINNAMON SMOOTHIE

Blueberries love cinnamon. Both are powerful sources of antioxidants, plus wild blueberries have even more antioxidants than regular blueberries. The hemp seeds, sometimes called hemp hearts, add plant-based omega-3s and a mild nuttiness that seamlessly blends into this smoothie. This smoothie is an excellent source of protein, fiber, potassium, vitamin B6, folate, vitamin E, and iron.

MIND foods: Berries, beans

Yield: 1 serving | **Time:** 5 minutes

½ cup cold unsweetened soy milk
1 seedless mandarin orange, peeled
½ teaspoon vanilla extract
1 teaspoon hemp seeds

½ teaspoon ground cinnamon
1 cup frozen wild blueberries
1 medium frozen ripe banana, broken
  into 3–4 pieces

1. Add the ingredients to a blender in the order listed and blend on high for 30–60 seconds, until smooth. Enjoy immediately.

Notes: For conventional blenders, add liquid first to help the blades spin more easily. Do the reverse for inverted blenders, sometimes called "personal blenders," with a blade and base that screws onto the top of the cup (for example, Nutribullet).

> **Nutrition:** 350 calories, 820 mg omega-3s, 1 g saturated fat, 10 g protein, 69 g carbohydrates, 12 g fiber, 0 g added sugars, 940 mg potassium, 0.7 mg vitamin B6, 90 mcg folate, 0 mcg vitamin B12, 40 mg choline, 320 mcg lutein

GOLDEN SUNSHINE SMOOTHIE

There are so many bright, golden-hued fruits, vegetables, and even spices in this powerful anti-inflammatory smoothie. Vitamin A from carrots, Vitamin C from mandarin oranges, both vitamins A and C from mango, and antioxidants from turmeric. This smoothie is rich in protein, fiber, potassium, vitamin B6, folate, vitamin E, and iron.

MIND foods: More vegetables, beans

Yield: 1 serving | **Time:** 10–15 minutes

½ cup cold unsweetened soy milk
1 seedless mandarin orange, peeled
zest from 1 lemon
2 teaspoons lemon juice
1 medium carrot, peeled and cut into 3
  to 4 big chunks

1 teaspoon chopped peeled fresh
  ginger
¼ level teaspoon ground turmeric
5–10 twists freshly ground pepper
1 medium frozen ripe banana, broken
  into 3–4 pieces
½ cup frozen mango chunks

1. Add the ingredients to a blender in the order listed and blend on high for 1–2 minutes until smooth and the carrot is fully integrated. Transfer to a 16- to 20-ounce glass. Enjoy immediately.

Notes: The carrot in this has the potential to be gritty if not fully blended. Note that lemons come in different sizes; if yours gives you less zest, the smoothie will still work. Take care to only zest the outermost lemon skin and none of the bitter white pith. If your smoothie is bitter, add a tiny pinch of salt to counteract the bitterness and bring out the sweetness.

Substitution options: If you don't have fresh ginger, it is also sold frozen in 1-teaspoon cubes. Alternatively, use ground ginger at a third of the amount called for (⅓ teaspoon in this recipe). Similarly, if you don't have ground turmeric, use three times the amount of fresh grated turmeric (1½ teaspoons in this recipe).

Nutrition: 300 calories, 300 mg omega-3s, 1 g saturated fat, 10 g protein, 63 g carbohydrates, 9 g fiber, 0 g added sugars, 1230 mg potassium, 0.8 mg vitamin B6, 120 mcg folate, 0 mcg vitamin B12, 40 mg choline, 350 mcg lutein

MACA MOCHA SMOOTHIE

Is it a smoothie, a morning mocha, or a milkshake? Take your pick. The bold flavors of coffee and cacao stand up to the earthiness of walnuts and are rounded out with the nuttiness of maca, a root vegetable from Peru related to (but tasting nothing like) broccoli. Note that coffee and cacao are natural sources of caffeine, so this is best enjoyed in the morning, or even adjusted with decaf coffee if you are sensitive to caffeine. This smoothie is an excellent source of protein, fiber, potassium, and vitamin B6, a good source of iron and folate, with plenty of plant-based omega-3s from walnuts.

MIND foods: Nuts

Yield: 1 serving | **Time:** 5 minutes

½ cup cold unsweetened soy milk
½ teaspoon vanilla extract
½ cup Americano (espresso + water), cold brew, or regular coffee
2 tablespoons walnut pieces

2 medjool dates, seedless
1 teaspoon maca powder
1 teaspoon cacao powder
1 medium frozen ripe banana, broken into 3-4 pieces

1. Add the ingredients to a blender in the order listed and blend on high for 1 to 1½ minutes, or until smooth. Transfer to a 16-ounce glass. Enjoy immediately.

Notes: Maca is a malty and nutty-tasting root vegetable, and the powder is available in health stores or online. Navitas is a popular brand. If you don't have a frozen ripe banana on hand, use a fresh ripe banana plus 2 large ice cubes (or 4–6 regular ice cubes)

Substitution options: If cacao powder (a less processed form of cocoa) is not available, use cocoa powder. Soy milk adds plant protein but can be swapped with other plant or animal milks.

Nutrition: 430 calories, 1370 mg omega-3s, 2 g saturated fat, 12 g protein, 74 g carbohydrates, 10 g fiber, 0 g added sugars, 1230 mg potassium, 0.7 mg vitamin B6, 70 mcg folate, 0 mcg vitamin B12, 30 mg choline, 40 mcg lutein

Small Plates

BERRY PARFAIT

This isn't your average parfait. The strawberries and creamy yogurt are the star of the show, but the luscious yet judiciously used prune puree is a sweet surprise with the mouthfeel of a chocolate swirl and a delightful base note. Enjoy this layered parfait any time for a good source of protein, polyphenols, and more. This dish is high in protein, fiber, vitamin E, calcium, and potassium, and a good source of iron, vitamin B6, folate, vitamin B12, and choline.

MIND foods: Berries, nuts

Yield: 1½ cups | **Time:** 10 minutes

PRUNE PUREE INGREDIENTS

½ cup tightly packed prunes
6 tablespoons hot water

INGREDIENTS

½ cup Greek yogurt
1 tablespoon creamy peanut butter
½ teaspoon pure vanilla extract
pinch of Diamond Crystal kosher salt

3 tablespoons Prune Puree
⅓ cup sliced strawberries
½ cup blueberries
3 tablespoons whole almonds

1. To make the prune puree, add the prunes to a mini food processor set to puree. Puree until smooth, adding the hot water slowly in small amounts or it'll splash out. Pause as needed to scrape down sides and bottom of bowl. You will have extra as this recipe makes about 2/3 cup. Store extra in an airtight container in the refrigerator for up to 4 weeks. See notes on uses.

2. In a small bowl, mix together the yogurt, peanut butter, vanilla extract, and salt.

3. In a 2-cup mason jar or glass, layer in ⅓ cup of the yogurt mixture, followed by 1½ tablespoons prune puree, half the strawberries, half the blueberries, and 2 tablespoons of almonds.

Repeat layering in the same order with remaining the yogurt, 1½ tablespoons prune puree, strawberries, blueberries, and almonds. Enjoy or cover and refrigerate for the following day.

Notes: You'll have extra prune puree from this recipe. Use it for a touch of natural sweetness and benefit from a boost of polyphenols and fiber, whether in oatmeal, swirled into yogurt, or added to marinades, dressings, and sauces. Try it in the Vegan Strawberry Yogurt (page 175), Creamy No-Cook PB&J Mousse (page 233) recipes.

Nutrition: 560 calories, 90 mg omega-3s, 3 g saturated fat, 28 g protein, 53 g carbohydrates, 12 g fiber, 0 g added sugars, 980 mg potassium, 0.3 mg vitamin B6, 60 mcg folate, 0.3 mcg vitamin B12, 50 mg choline, 120 mcg lutein

SPICY GREENS & EGG TOAST

The green sauce used in this recipe is meant to be punch-in-your-face spicy, inspired by zhoug sauce, a cilantro-forward spicy sauce thought to have origins in Yemen. For less of a burn, omit the jalapeño, or take it up a notch by adding the whole jalapeño. This breakfast toast balances the heat of the sauce with cooling yogurt, earthy whole grain toast, and mild eggs. It is an excellent source of protein, vitamin B12, and choline, and a good source of fiber, vitamin E, iron, vitamin B6, and folate.

MIND foods: Leafy greens, more vegetables, whole grains, olive oil
Yield: 1 breakfast toast and ⅔ cup sauce | **Time:** 20 minutes

GREEN SAUCE

2 cups packed fresh cilantro leaves and stems
½ cup packed fresh parsley leaves and stems
2 tablespoons fresh mint leaves
2 tablespoons avocado oil
1 clove garlic

1 tablespoon fresh lime juice
¼ teaspoon Diamond Crystal kosher salt
½ fresh medium jalapeño (optional)
½ teaspoon ground cumin
⅛ teaspoon ground cardamom
½ teaspoon gochugaru

EGGS AND TOAST

1 slice whole wheat toast
1 teaspoon olive oil
1 egg
2 teaspoons green sauce

pinch of gochugaru
1 tablespoon strained yogurt (e.g., Greek or Icelandic)

1. Trim browned cilantro stems and any thick parsley stems, but keep most of the stems.

2. To make the green sauce, in a mini food processor, add the fresh herbs, avocado oil, garlic, lime juice, salt, and jalapeño, if using. Set to chop and pulse in 2-second intervals until the mixture looks like wet cut grass. Pause the processor as needed to scrape down the sides and bottom, 1–2 minutes total. Transfer to a medium bowl and stir in cumin, cardamom, and gochugaru.

3. Toast the bread in a toaster.

4. Heat the olive oil in a small nonstick pan over medium heat, 1 minute. Add the egg and cook until whites are almost set, 2–3 minutes. Break the yolk with a spatula or fork and gently flatten. Flip and cook for 1 minute. Set aside.

5. Spread strained yogurt on toast. Top with 2 teaspoons of green sauce, dotted evenly on top of yogurt. Top with flattened egg. Sprinkle with gochugaru.

Notes: As an alternative to a mini-food processor for the green sauce, mince fresh herbs and garlic ingredients with a chef's knife and stir in salt and spices in a medium bowl.

For quicker mornings, make the green sauce a day ahead so it's ready to go. Store it in an airtight container in the refrigerator for up to a week. Leftover sauce can be added to pastas, used as a sandwich spread, or drizzled on top of scrambled eggs.

> **Nutrition:** 240 calories, 130 mg omega-3s, 3 g saturated fat, 13 g protein, 20 g carbohydrates, 3 g fiber, 2 g added sugars, 230 mg potassium, 0.2 mg vitamin B6, 50 mcg folate, 0.6 mcg vitamin B12, 160 mg choline, 390 mcg lutein

PB&J STEEL CUT OATS

This warm bowl of simple goodness is a grown-up PB&J. It combines the beloved flavors of peanut butter and jelly sandwiches, but uses whole nuts and berries over steel cut oats. This dish is rich in protein and fiber, and provides a good source of vitamin E, iron, vitamin B6, and folate.

MIND foods: Berries, nuts, whole grains

Yield: 1 bowl | **Time:** 30 minutes

1½ cups water
¼ cup dry steel cut oats
2 pinches of Diamond Crystal kosher salt
1 tablespoon peanut butter

½ cup sliced strawberries
½ cup fresh raspberries
1 tablespoon peanuts, chopped

1. Bring water to a boil in a medium saucepan. Stir in oats and salt and reduce heat to low. Simmer uncovered 25 minutes, stirring occasionally until at a loose porridge consistency. It will continue to thicken as it cools.

2. Turn heat off and stir in peanut butter.

3. To serve, add oats to a bowl and top with strawberries, raspberries, and peanuts.

Substitution options: Try using different nut butters, nuts, and berries as variations. Chopped apples, hemp hearts, and chia seeds would all make great toppings.

Level-up: The steel cut oats and peanut butter can be made in advance and in larger batches in order to get to breakfast faster. If the mixture seems too thick, it can be warmed up with a little additional water or milk to loosen it.

Nutrition: 325 calories, 100 mg omega-3s, 2 g saturated fat, 12 g protein, 38 g carbohydrates, 9 g fiber, 0 g added sugars, 420 mg potassium, 0.2 mg vitamin B6, 70 mcg folate, 0 mcg vitamin B12, 40 mg choline, 120 mcg lutein

BERRY FONIO

This is a one-bowl, 5-minute meal to get you fueled, stat. Perfect for when you're short on time and need more ideas for how to add whole grains to your day. This dish works as a quick breakfast, snack, or light lunch. It is an excellent source of protein, fiber, vitamin E, iron, and folate, and a good source of potassium and vitamin B6.

MIND foods: Berries, nuts, whole grains, olive oil

Yield: 1 (1¼-cup) serving | **Time:** 5 minutes

¼ cup fonio
1 cup unsweetened soy milk
1 teaspoon olive oil
⅛ teaspoon Diamond Crystal kosher salt

½ cup sliced strawberries
½ cup blueberries
1 tablespoon whole almonds

1. In a medium microwave-safe bowl, mix together fonio, soy milk, olive oil, and salt.

2. Cover and microwave for 2 minutes. Stir. Cover and cook for an additional 2 minutes. Rest covered for an additional 3 minutes. Uncover and stir.

3. Top with strawberries, blueberries, and almonds.

Substitution options: Try other combinations of fruits, vegetables, and nuts. For example, roasted diced sweet potatoes, cinnamon, and pecans; chopped apples and walnuts; or fresh raspberries, blackberries, and cashews.

Nutrition: 465 calories, 530 mg omega-3s, 2 g saturated fat, 19 g protein, 60 g carbohydrates, 6 g fiber, 0 g added sugars, 720 mg potassium, 0.3 mg vitamin B6, 90 mcg folate, 0 mcg vitamin B12, 30 mg choline, 80 mcg lutein

SMOKED TROUT TOAST

Smoked trout is familiar and reminds me of tuna, yet has a milder flavor profile that allows it to melt into this spread seamlessly. This small plate is savory, fresh, and satisfying. The smoked trout spread could easily do

double-duty on its own as a veggie dip. This dish is rich in protein, vitamin D, and vitamin B12, and provides a good source of fiber, vitamin E, and vitamin B6.

MIND foods: More vegetables, seafood, whole grains

Yield: 1 toast with 3 tablespoons spread (~⅔ cup smoked trout spread total) | **Time:** 7 minutes

1 slice whole grain toast
3 tablespoons Smoked Trout Spread
    (page 167)
freshly ground black pepper, to taste

1. Spread 3 tablespoons of the smoked trout spread on toast and top with extra radishes, cucumbers, green onion or parsley, if using. Finish with freshly ground black pepper.

SMOKED TROUT SPREAD

⅓ cup reduced fat Greek yogurt
1½ teaspoons fresh lemon juice
1 stalk green onion, trimmed and
    sliced, plus more to garnish
    (optional)
¼ teaspoon soy sauce
½ medium radish, finely diced, plus
    more to garnish (optional)

1-inch piece English cucumber, peel
on, finely diced, plus more to garnish
    (optional)
1 teaspoon packed fresh flat leaf
    parsley, leaves only, chopped, plus
    more to garnish (optional)
1 (3.9-ounce) tin smoked trout in oil,
    drained

1. In a medium bowl, stir together all smoked trout spread ingredients except trout until well combined. Add smoked trout and gently stir it into the mix until just combined.

2. Spread 3 tablespoons of the smoked trout spread on toast and top with extra radishes, cucumbers, green onion, and parsley, if using. Finish with freshly ground black pepper.

> **Nutrition:** 185 calories, 450 mg omega-3s, 1 g saturated fat, 16 g protein, 20 g carbohydrates, 3 g fiber, 2 g added sugars, 310 mg potassium, 0.2 mg vitamin B6, 30 mcg folate, 1.5 mcg vitamin B12, 40 mg choline, 90 mcg lutein

MINI FRITTATAS

The secret to packing a ton of flavor into these little bites is a team effort between the sautéed mushrooms and sun-dried tomatoes. These little guys are freezer-friendly, so you can make a batch and enjoy it anytime. A serving of these frittatas provides an excellent source of protein, vitamin D, vitamin B12, choline, and iron.

MIND foods: More vegetables, seafood, olive oil

Yield: 8 (3-frittata) servings | **Time:** 30–35 minutes

8 large eggs
½ cup Greek yogurt
2 tablespoons olive oil
1 anchovy fillet, from tin or jar packed in oil
8 baby portobello mushrooms, roughly chopped
¼ cup chopped white onion

¼ teaspoon Diamond Crystal kosher salt, divided
½ cup chopped asparagus
¼ teaspoon gochugaru
½ cup packed sun-dried tomatoes packed in oil, minced
1½ teaspoons Italian seasoning
freshly ground black pepper, to taste

1. Preheat the oven to 325°F.

2. In a large mixing bowl, blend eggs and yogurt together, 10 seconds. Set aside.

3. Heat olive oil in a medium nonstick pan, 1–2 minutes. Mash anchovy into the olive oil to "melt" it into the oil, 30 seconds.

4. Add mushrooms, onion, and half of salt to pan, stirring occasionally until mushrooms are reduced, 5 minutes.

5. Add asparagus and half of remaining salt and cook for another 4 minutes. Stir in gochugaru and remaining salt. Turn heat off.

6. Place silicone mini muffin pan on a sheet pan. Distribute a teaspoon of the mushroom-onion mix into each cup. Next, distribute about ½ teaspoon of the minced sun-dried tomatoes into each cup. Top each cup with about 1 tablespoon of egg-yogurt mixture. Finally, sprinkle Italian seasoning evenly across cups and grind fresh pepper on top.

7. Roast for 10 minutes, rotate pan, and return to oven for 5 minutes.

8. Enjoy right away, cool for 15 minutes then refrigerate in an airtight container for 3–4 days (reheat in microwave for 15–30 seconds), or cool for 15 minutes then place entire pan in the freezer for 1 hour to flash freeze, then pop mini-frittatas out and store in a freezer-safe container in the freezer for 1–3 months (reheat in microwave 30–60 seconds.)

Notes: Eggs love to stick to muffin tins, but they pop right out of silicone muffin pans, which also do a better job of insulating the eggs from heat, for gentler cooking.

> **Nutrition:** 160 calories, 80 mg omega-3s, 2 g saturated fat, 10 g protein, 6 g carbohydrates, 2 g fiber, 0 g added sugars, 200 mg potassium, 0.1 mg vitamin B6, 40 mcg folate, 0.7 mcg vitamin B12, 160 mg choline, 280 mcg lutein

OPEN-FACED OMELET WITH SMOKED TROUT

So much flavor in such little time. Smoked trout adds depth without being overly fishy. This quick breakfast will get you a serving of greens, extra veggies, and brain-healthy choline from the eggs plus omega-3s from the fish. Did I mention it's quick and delicious? It's the best of both worlds. This dish is packed with protein, vitamin B12, and choline, and provides a good source of vitamin D, iron, and potassium.

MIND foods: Leafy greens, more vegetables, seafood, olive oil
Yield: 1 large omelet or 2 medium omelets | **Time:** 15 minutes

2 large eggs
1 tablespoon unsweetened soy milk
1 (3.9-ounce) tin smoked trout in oil, drained
2 teaspoons olive oil, plus more if pan is dry

½ cup grape tomatoes, halved
pinch of Diamond Crystal kosher salt, divided
2 cups packed dark leafy baby greens (e.g., baby kale, baby spinach)

1. In a medium bowl, whisk together eggs and milk. Add smoked trout and use gentle pressure to break into almond-sized flakes. Set aside. Wash hands.

2. Heat olive oil in a 10-inch nonstick pan, 1–2 minutes. Add tomatoes and a half pinch of salt, shaking pan occasionally until tomatoes wilt. If pan becomes dry, add an additional teaspoon of olive oil.

3. Add leafy greens and final half-pinch of salt, cover for 30 seconds, then stir uncovered until wilted but still bright green, 1–2 minutes.

4. Pour egg mixture over pan, tilting to spread it evenly. Cover and cook 2–3 minutes, or until egg whites have just set.

5. For 1 large omelet, slide the omelet onto a large plate or fold it over as it slides out of the pan. For 2 two medium omelets, use a non-metal spatula to break it into two even semicircles before plating. It can also go from stovetop to the table in the pan, be divided into four "slices," and used to top whole grain toast.

Notes: This is very flavorful on its own, but some people may enjoy an additional dollop of plain Greek yogurt, Green Sauce (page 163), or chili crisp on top.

> **Nutrition:** 220 calories, 80 mg omega-3s, 3 g saturated fat, 17 g protein, 5 g carbohydrates, 2 g fiber, 0 g added sugars, 490 mg potassium, 0.1 mg vitamin B6, 30 mcg folate, 0.6 mcg vitamin B12, 150 mg choline, 230 mcg lutein

Snacks

NO-BAKE CHEWY GRANOLA BALLS

Make once, enjoy for days (or longer if you stash them in the freezer). Each one of these granola balls is about half a regular granola bar, so you can decide if you feel like popping 1, 2, or 3, depending on your hunger level. These sweet bites are a fun way to eat more whole grains, nuts, berries, and omega-3s.

MIND foods: Berries, nuts, whole grains

Yield: 32 (1-tablespoon) servings | **Time:** 20 minutes

DATE PASTE

2 cups packed medjool dates
2–3 cups water, for boiling dates

½ cup cool water

GRANOLA BALLS

1 cup Date Paste
1½ cups rolled oats
2 tablespoons chia seeds
¼ cup peanut butter

1 cup dried wild blueberries,
    unsweetened if available
¾ cup roughly chopped almonds
1 tablespoon toasted sesame seeds
½ teaspoon flaky sea salt (e.g., Maldon
    sea salt flakes)

1. Place dates in a medium pot and add water until just covered. Bring to boil, and boil for 10 minutes. Remove from heat, drain.

2. Add dates and ½ cup of cool water to a mini food processor and set to puree. Pulse until smooth, pausing to open the lid and scrape down the sides with a spatula as needed. Transfer 1 cup of date paste to a storage container. Date, label, and refrigerate for another use. 1 cup of date paste will remain in the food processor.

3. Add rolled oats, chia seeds, and peanut butter to the mini food processor and set to chop. Pulse until the mixture has a sand-like texture and sticks together when pinched. Pause as needed to open the lid and scrape down the sides with a spatula. Transfer mixture to a large bowl.

4. To the large bowl with the date-oat mixture, add wild blueberries and chopped almonds. Stir gently to incorporate, or put on disposable food prep gloves and massage the ingredients together.

5. If it's not holding together well, freeze for at least 20 minutes so it sets a little but isn't hard.

6. Scoop a level tablespoon and roll into a ball, then transfer to a 9½ x 13-inch sheet pan or larger. Continue scooping the remaining mixture and add to the sheet pan in a single layer.

7. Sprinkle the balls with sesame seeds and roll them around to pick up sesame seeds that didn't stick. Repeat with the flaky salt.

Notes: Store these in an airtight container, separating layers with parchment paper if desired. Keep for 1 week in the refrigerator or 2 months in the freezer. To eat from frozen, let them thaw at room temperature for a few minutes or until they have some give when pinched.

This recipe makes more date paste than you need for the granola bars. You can use leftovers in Turkey Chili (page 196) or Doenjang Salmon Lettuce Wraps (page 215).

Replacing Sugar: When replacing white granulated sugar, replace it 1:1. When replacing maple syrup or honey, use twice the date paste in a 2:1 ratio.

Substitution options: Try tahini or sunflower seed butter for a nut-free alternative to peanut butter.

Level-up: Date paste can be made in advance. If you have the patience, reduce food waste by reserving ½ cup of the cooking liquid to use instead of the cool water, but let it cool first or the steam will create unwanted pressure in the food processor; plus, the heat will cook the oats. Another alternative is to soak the dates in room temperature water for 2 hours and drain, but save ½ cup of this liquid to use right away.

Nutrition: 80 calories, 120 mg omega-3s, 0 g saturated fat, 2 g protein, 12 g carbohydrates, 2 g fiber, 0 g added sugars, 120 mg potassium, 0 mg vitamin B6, 10 mcg folate, 0 mcg vitamin B12, 10 mg choline, 20 mcg lutein

GINGER-CITRUS VITALITY BITES

When you want an inflammation-busting bite bursting with bold flavors and nutrients, make a batch of these little bites. They're only little in size. They're large on bioactives and powerful spices like turmeric.

MIND foods: Nuts, whole grains, olive oil
Yield: 35 (1-teaspoon bite) servings | **Time:** 20 minutes

zest from 2 large lemons, divided
zest from 2 medium mandarin
    oranges, divided
½ teaspoon + 2 pinches of Diamond
    Crystal kosher salt, divided
1 cup packed medjool dates
1 tablespoon fresh lemon juice
½ cup walnuts
½ cup unsalted cashews

¼ cup chia seeds
¼ cup oats
3 teaspoons ground ginger
2 teaspoons ground turmeric
¼ teaspoon freshly ground black
    pepper
¼ teaspoon ground cardamom
1 teaspoon olive oil

1. Set aside half of the lemon zest (2 tablespoons) and half of the mandarin orange zest (1 tablespoon) in a small bowl. Separately, set aside 2 pinches of salt in a small bowl.

2. Combine the remaining ingredients in a mini-food processor and set to chop. Pulse 10–15 times, in 1-second intervals, until mixture is integrated and sticks together when pinched. Pause to scrape down sides and bottom of mixer as needed.

3. Spoon about 1 teaspoon of mixture at a time and roll between palms into ¾-inch balls. It's OK if they're not all uniform. Set them aside on a rimmed sheet pan. Be mindful that the turmeric in these can stain.

4. Sprinkle bites with reserved 2 pinches of salt, 2 tablespoons lemon zest, and 1 tablespoon of orange zest. Gently shake the baking sheet to coat.

5. Transfer to a storage container. These will keep in the refrigerator for up to a week, or in the freezer for 2–3 months. They can be enjoyed directly from the freezer without any thawing time.

Notes: These little bites are intense and bold. If it's too much for your palate, scale back on the turmeric, ginger, and lemon zest by half, add one more date, and sprinkle an additional ⅛ teaspoon of salt over your final product. The flavor is also less intense the colder they are, so you may try them straight from the freezer.

OVEN-DRIED CITRUS CIRCLES

The ingredients for this recipe are mandarin oranges and time. Your patience will be rewarded. The drying process concentrates the flavors and makes the thin rind of mandarins edible and pleasantly bitter against the sweetness of the fruit. Eat this on their own or add to salads, mocktails, and desserts like the Almond Citrus Chocolate Bites (page 232).

Yield: 6 (4- to 8-circle) servings | **Time:** 60 minutes

8 cold mandarin oranges

1. Preheat the oven to 200°F.

2. Use a mandoline to create even ¼-inch mandarin slices or thinner. You'll get 3 good slices and up to 3 OK slices from each mandarin. The colder they are, the more easily they will slice. If you have particularly juicy mandarins, you may get less. Any leftover mandarin parts can be juiced to enjoy on the spot or stored for a later use.

3. Line a large sheet pan with a silicone baking mat. Arrange mandarin orange slices in a single layer. Dry in oven for 45 minutes, checking on them and rotating the pan every 15 minutes. For the final 15 minutes, check at 10 minutes and return the pan to the oven for the final 5 minutes with the heat off. At each check, set aside any citrus circles with partial browning or any singed edges. They are OK to eat but shouldn't go back in the oven.

4. Transfer the citrus circles to a wire rack to cool completely, then store in an airtight container in a cool dry place for up to a year.

Notes: Oven temperatures are variable and many start at 200°F. If your oven goes lower, that will provide a nice gentle drying but will take longer. If you have a convection setting, use it.

Regardless, keep an eye on your citrus circles so they don't burn. The regular check-ins written into the recipe help with this but are also functional—the act of opening the oven door brings the temperature down.

Try snacking on these on their own, or dip them in dark chocolate and sprinkle with crushed nuts or sea salt for a festive treat. They can also be added to mocktails or used to decorate baked goods.

Substitution options: This method will work on any citrus, though total dry time may vary. Try this with lemons, oranges, grapefruit, and more.

> **Nutrition:** 40 calories, 10 mg omega-3s, 0 g saturated fat, 1 g protein, 10 g carbohydrates, 1 g fiber, 0 g added sugars, 130 mg potassium, 0.1 mg vitamin B6, 10 mcg folate, 0 mcg vitamin B12, 10 mg choline, 110 mcg lutein

VEGAN STRAWBERRY YOGURT

If you're curious about trying a plant-based yogurt alternative, need one because you're allergic or sensitive to dairy, or are seeking something lactose-free, this is for you. This light snack is a good source of protein, iron, and folate.

MIND foods: Berries, beans

Yield: 2 (⅔-cup) servings | **Time:** 10 minutes

1 cup whole strawberries
1 cup soft silken tofu
½ teaspoon lemon zest
1 teaspoon pure vanilla extract

3 tablespoons Prune Puree (page 162)
2 pinches of Diamond Crystal kosher salt

1. Blend all ingredients until smooth.

Notes: Try the Prune Puree in the Creamy No-Cook PB&J Mousse (page 233) and the Berry Parfait (page 162).

Substitution options: Try this with other berries!

BEET-PICKLED EGGS

The Pennsylvania Dutch are credited with introducing the United States to beet-pickled eggs, though I was introduced to them by a recipe contest challenging dietitians to create their own take on this pretty-in-pink dish. This is an update to my entry. Yes there is a waiting period for this dish, but your wait will be rewarded with pink-haloed eggs with a tangy bite. Each pickled egg is an excellent source of vitamin B12 and choline and a good source of protein and folate.

MIND foods: More vegetables

Yield: 6 (1-beet-pickled egg) servings | **Time:** 30 minutes, plus 24–48 hours to chill

6 eggs

liquid from 1 (15-ounce) can sliced beets

1 cup apple cider vinegar

1 medjool date, minced

1 teaspoon Diamond Crystal kosher salt

1 teaspoon whole black peppercorn (optional)

1 teaspoon whole white peppercorn (optional)

1 teaspoon whole coriander seed (optional)

½ teaspoon mustard seeds (optional)

6–12 ice cubes (optional)

½ cup sliced red onions (optional)

1. In a medium pot on high, cover eggs with water and bring to a boil. Once boiling, turn heat off, cover, and set a timer for 11 minutes.

2. In a small saucepan over medium heat, add the beet juice, apple cider vinegar, minced medjool date, salt, and, if using, the whole peppercorns and seeds and bring to a boil. Reduce heat and simmer for 5 minutes.

3. In a medium bowl, combine the ice cubes with a cup of water to make an ice bath. When the eggs are ready, transfer them to the

ice bath with a slotted spoon. When cool enough to handle, peel, rinsing any small shell bits off by dipping eggs back in the water as needed. Put shells in a discard bowl.

4. Into a tall 3- to 4-cup heat-resistant jar with lid such as a mason jar, layer the peeled eggs and red onion slices throughout. Pour the hot beet juice mixture over eggs. Cover and refrigerate for 24–48 hours.

Notes: If your eggs aren't fully submerged, add vinegar and water in a 1:1 ratio until they are covered. If there's room, feel free to toss in a few beet slices (from the canned beets) or more red onion into your pickling jar; otherwise, save the beets for the Beets & Berries Barley Salad (page 185) or Ruby Red Veggie-Veggie Dip (page 177). Enjoy the eggs on their own, or slice and add to sandwiches and salads. The pickled red onions are also delicious and can be added like a relish to sandwiches, avocado toast, chicken, or fish.

Nutrition: 105 calories, 30 mg omega-3s, 1 g saturated fat, 6 g protein, 7 g carbohydrates, 1 g fiber, 0 g added sugars, 210 mg potassium, 0.1 mg vitamin B6, 40 mcg folate, 0.5 mcg vitamin B12, 130 mg choline, 160 mcg lutein

RUBY RED VEGGIE-VEGGIE DIP

My husband calls this veggie-veggie dip because we love it with veggies and it's made with veggies. I hope you enjoy it as much as we do. It also works as a sandwich spread, on top of a baked potato, or as an anchoring sauce when plating roasted veggies, grilled chicken, or roasted fish. Each serving is a good source of fiber.

MIND foods: More vegetables, beans, olive oil

Yield: 7½ (¼-cup) servings | **Time:** 5 minutes

1 clove garlic, roughly chopped
1 (15-ounce) can cannellini beans, drained and rinsed until foaming stops
⅓ cup sliced beets

2 tablespoons fresh lemon juice
1½ teaspoons water
½ teaspoon Diamond Crystal kosher salt
¼ teaspoon gochugaru

⅛ teaspoon white pepper
2 tablespoons olive oil

1 teaspoon olive oil, to garnish (optional)
fresh flat-leaf parsley, leaves only, chopped, to garnish (optional)

1. Combine all ingredients in a mini food processor and set to puree. Pulse until smooth, scraping down sides as needed. If eating right away, transfer to a serving bowl and garnish with a drizzle of best quality olive oil and fresh parsley, if using.

2. Otherwise, refrigerate in an airtight container for 4–5 days.

Notes: This recipe uses canned beets for convenience, but you can swap in freshly roasted beets. If you find the flavor of roasted beets to be strong, then you may prefer the milder flavor of canned beets.

Substitution options: Any white bean will work in this recipe. Cannellini beans can be swapped for navy or great northern beans, for example. To reduce spiciness, reduce the gochugaru or replace with paprika.

Nutrition: 80 calories, 60 mg omega-3s, 1 g saturated fat, 3 g protein, 9 g carbohydrates, 3 g fiber, 0 g added sugars, 190 mg potassium, 0.1 mg vitamin B6, 20 mcg folate, 0 mcg vitamin B12, 15 mg choline, 10 mcg lutein

CUKE & CUMIN YOGURT DIP

You'll love the cooling and refreshing yet savory flavor of this dip, which is inspired by both tzatziki and raita, two yogurt-based condiments. Yogurt and cucumber are often found in both, garlic more often in the Greek tzatziki and cumin more often in the Indian raita. They each have several variations in their own right. This one isn't quite either, but it owes everything to both. Each serving is a good source of vitamin B12.

MIND foods: More vegetables, olive oil
Yield: 6 (¼-cup) servings | **Time:** 20 minutes

6 inches Korean cucumber

2 pinches + ¼ teaspoon Diamond Crystal kosher salt, divided

1 clove garlic, minced
1 tablespoon chopped fresh mint
   leaves
1 cup Greek yogurt

1 tablespoon fresh lemon juice
1 teaspoon ground cumin
1½ teaspoons olive oil

1. Peel the cucumber and grate on the largest shredding holes. Set over a fine mesh strainer placed over a medium bowl, 15 minutes. Press to release more liquid.

2. Work 2 pinches of salt into the garlic, mashing it into a paste with the back of a knife or the side of a glass. Or, use a mortar and pestle, 1 minute.

3. Stack mint leaves and roll them together to make them easier to handle. Slice crosswise into thin ribbons.

4. In a medium bowl, stir together the yogurt, garlic paste, lemon juice, cumin, and ¼ teaspoon salt. Squeeze a handful of the grated cucumbers between your palms to release as much liquid as possible before adding to the yogurt mixture. Repeat with the rest of the cucumber. Add the mint and gently stir everything together. Drizzle with olive oil just before serving.

5. Serving suggestions: Serve as a dip with vegetables such as cauliflower, broccoli, bell peppers, carrots, and more; as a spread on pita bread topped with tomatoes; or dolloped next to some chana masala and whole wheat naan.

Notes: The liquid that drains from the grated cucumbers is refreshing. It's not a lot, but feel free to drink it for a little extra nutrition rather than discard it.

Nutrition: 40 calories, 20 mg omega-3s, 0 g saturated fat, 4 g protein, 3 g carbohydrates, 0 g fiber, 0 g added sugars, 110 mg potassium, 0.1 mg vitamin B6, 10 mcg folate, 0.3 mcg vitamin B12, 10 mg choline, 30 mcg lutein

BLACK BEAN DIP

This savory black bean dip has just the right balance of tart, spice, and everything nice. Use your best olive oil. Each serving is a good source of fiber and folate with a modest amount of plant-based protein too.

MIND foods: Beans, olive oil

Yield: Makes 6 (¼-cup) servings | **Time:** 10 minutes

1 tablespoon extra-virgin olive oil

1 tablespoon fig balsamic vinegar

2 tablespoons fresh lime juice

1 teaspoon Diamond Crystal kosher salt

½ teaspoon ground cumin

½ teaspoon gochugaru

1 small clove garlic

1 (15-ounce) can black beans, drained and rinsed

1. Add all ingredients to a mini food processor in the order listed, which will help avoid splattering. Set to puree and pulse until smooth. Transfer to a serving bowl.

2. Serve with carrot sticks, radish wedges, grape tomatoes, or whole wheat pita chips.

Notes: If the dip is thicker than you prefer, stir in a tablespoon of warm water at a time until desired consistency is reached. To avoid splatter, either stream the liquid in slowly to the mini-processor, or transfer the bean dip to a medium mixing bowl before adding liquid.

Substitution options: If fig balsamic vinegar is unavailable, use regular balsamic vinegar.

Nutrition: 85 calories, 90 mg omega-3s, 0 g saturated fat, 4 g protein, 13 g carbohydrates, 5 g fiber, 0 g added sugars, 190 mg potassium, 0.1 mg vitamin B6, 60 mcg folate, 0 mcg vitamin B12, 20 mg choline, 1 mcg lutein

CRUNCHY SPICED CHICKPEAS

Crunchy spiced chickpeas are a healthy snack that delivers on crunch and flavor. You can make crunchy chickpeas that stay crunchy right in your own kitchen. The secret is a low and slow roast. Thankfully, most of that time is inactive. Each serving is an excellent source of fiber and a good source of protein, iron, and folate.

MIND foods: Beans, olive oil

Yield: 5 (⅓-cup) servings | **Time:** 2 hours

2 (15-ounce) cans chickpeas, drained, rinsed

3 tablespoons olive oil

1 teaspoon Diamond Crystal kosher salt

2 teaspoons ground cumin

½ teaspoon garlic powder

½ teaspoon ground ginger

½ teaspoon gochugaru

½ teaspoon freshly ground black pepper

1. Drain and rinse chickpeas, swirling them in a colander under streaming water until they stop foaming. Lay the chickpeas in one layer between two towels and gently roll them. Spend a few minutes removing skins that have come loose. Don't worry about doing them all. Let them dry for 30 minutes. If the bottom towel is soaked, change it out.

2. Preheat the oven to 350°F for 15 minutes.

3. In a large bowl, combine all ingredients and toss to coat. Transfer chickpeas to a large rimmed sheet pan lined with a silicone mat, spreading them in one layer. Set the large bowl with remaining spice mix aside for later.

4. Roast for 45 minutes, opening the oven every 15 minutes to shake and rotate the pan. The chickpeas are done when they have lost 30–50 percent of their original size, are crunchy, and lightly browned but not dark. Watch them closely toward the end. The last 15 minutes may be split into 5-minute increments so that they don't overcook.

5. When the chickpeas are done, transfer them back to the large bowl with the remaining spice mix and swirl to coat. Add a teaspoon more oil if it seems dry. Transfer them back to the sheet pan to cool, at least 30 minutes. Transfer to an airtight container and store in a cool dry place for 4–5 days.

Notes: Snack on these anytime, or add them to salads or as a garnish to soups.

Level-up: Removing the skins, which hold some moisture, helps the chickpeas crisp up. If time and patience allow, remove all the skins. This is also a fun job for kitchen helpers (e.g., kids, friends, family).

Nutrition: 205 calories, 90 mg omega-3s, 1 g saturated fat, 7 g protein, 23 g carbohydrates, 7 g fiber, 0 g added sugars, 160 mg potassium, 0.1 mg vitamin B6, 50 mcg folate, 0 mcg vitamin B12, 40 mg choline, 10 mcg lutein

Salads

SUMMER KALE SALAD

We don't always think of kale as a summer vegetable, but it's available year round. The white nectarines are what make this kale salad summer-worthy. They provide a pop of crisp natural sweetness that adds a bright contrast to the hearty kale. Stone fruit like white nectarines are at their best in the summer. In other seasons, this salad works well with apples or pears. In a pinch, this salad also works well without fruit. It is rich in vitamin E and a good source of protein, fiber, calcium, and iron.

MIND foods: Leafy greens, more vegetables, olive oil

Yield: 4 (large salad) servings | **Time:** 15 to 20 minutes

8 cups loosely packed lacinato kale	1 white nectarine, cored and chopped
4 asparagus spears	1 tablespoon olive oil
2 pinches of Diamond Crystal kosher salt	¼ cup sliced almonds
1 large lemon, zested and juiced	

1. Remove the stems from kale. Roll leaves together and slice crosswise into thin strips. Transfer to a large bowl.

2. Trim the asparagus spears and use a Y-peeler to create long asparagus shavings. Alternatively, use a chef's knife to cut long, thin strips. Transfer to the large bowl with the kale.

3. Add the salt and lemon juice and massage until the kale just starts to wilt, 1–3 minutes. Don't overdo it.

4. Add the lemon zest, nectarine, and olive oil and toss to coat. Transfer to a serving bowl to serve family style. Garnish with sliced almonds just before serving.

Substitution options: Try this with a bunch of asparagus as the main green instead of kale. Use a Y-peeler to shave the asparagus into thin strips first. Make the rest of the salad as written.

Nutrition: 150 calories, 30 mg omega-3s, 1 g saturated fat, 7 g protein, 20 g carbohydrates, 5 g fiber, 0 g added sugars, 180 mg potassium, 0 mg vitamin B6, 14 mcg folate, 0 mcg vitamin B12, 7 mg choline, 120 mcg lutein

FLATBREAD SALAD

Fresh cucumbers and tomatoes are complemented by toasty bread chips and savory chicken in this riff on a Lebanese fattoush salad. This recipe makes smart use of convenient grocery-store rotisserie chicken and breathes new life into stale whole wheat flatbread to reduce food waste. This meal-sized savory salad is rich in protein, fiber, and vitamins B6 and B12. It also provides a good source of vitamin E, calcium, iron, potassium, vitamin B6, and choline.

MIND foods: Leafy greens, more vegetables, beans, whole grains, olive oil
Yield: 4 (large-salad servings) | **Time:** 15–20 minutes

1 piece stale whole wheat flatbread, torn into bite-sized pieces
1 medium vine-ripened tomato, cut into 8 wedges
2 tablespoons extra-virgin olive oil
2 tablespoons fresh lemon juice
1 pinch + ½ teaspoons Diamond Crystal kosher salt, divided
¼ teaspoon smoked ground paprika
2 pinches lemon pepper
1 pinch of five-spice powder
12 ounces chicken breast from store-bought rotisserie chicken

(unseasoned, when available), cut into bite-sized pieces or shredded
4 cups loosely packed leafy greens
1 medium carrot, peeled and chopped
6-inch Kirby cucumber, quartered and sliced
¼ cup canned chickpeas, rinsed and dried
1 stalk green onion, sliced
10 fresh mint leaves, hand-torn
freshly cracked black pepper to taste to garnish (optional)
additional olive oil, to garnish (optional)

1. Toast the bread in a toaster oven or in a dry pan until lightly browned. Set aside.

2. Sprinkle the cut sides of the tomatoes with a pinch of salt. Set aside.

3. To make the dressing, whisk together in a small bowl the olive oil, lemon juice, remaining salt, paprika, lemon pepper, and five-spice powder.

4. In a large bowl, combine the chicken, flatbread, and dressing and toss to coat. Add the remaining ingredients except tomatoes, and toss again. Transfer to salad bowls, top each bowl with a few freshly torn mint leaves, and finish with 2 tomato wedges and freshly cracked black pepper. If desired, add a final drizzle of olive oil to each bowl before eating.

Note: If Kirby cucumbers are unavailable, use any small-seed cucumber, including Korean, Persian, or English cucumbers.

Nutrition: 290 calories, 250 mg omega-3s, 2 g saturated fat, 30 g protein, 14 g carbohydrates, 7 g fiber, 0 g added sugars, 620 mg potassium, 0.5 mg vitamin B6, 30 mcg folate, 0.85 mcg vitamin B12, 90 mg choline, 140 mcg lutein

BEETS & BERRIES BARLEY SALAD

This is a hearty salad with filling barley, gently earthy beets, peppery arugula, bright strawberries, and balsamic vinegar, plus plenty of omega-3s from a full serving of walnuts per salad. The tiny bit of goat cheese goes a long way. This salad is great on its own but also works well with chicken or lean pork. It's an excellent source of protein, fiber, iron, and folate, and a good source of calcium, potassium, and vitamin B6.

MIND foods: Leafy greens, more vegetables, berries, nuts, whole grains, olive oil

Yield: 2 (2-cup) servings | **Time:** 15 minutes

1 cup drained sliced canned beets, chopped

2 teaspoons lemon juice, divided

2 teaspoons balsamic vinegar, divided

2 pinches Diamond Crystal kosher salt

1 cup cooked barley

2 cups packed baby arugula

½ cup strawberries, trimmed and sliced

½ cup walnuts, chopped

1 tablespoon olive oil, divided

2 teaspoons soft goat cheese, divided

1 pinch of freshly ground black pepper, divided, to taste

1. In a medium bowl, combine the beets, 1 teaspoon of lemon juice, 1 teaspoon of balsamic vinegar, and salt. Toss to coat and set aside.

2. Place cooked barley in a medium bowl, cover with a large plate, and microwave for 1 minute. Stir and repeat one more time if needed to warm through. Alternatively, make ½ cup dry barley according to package directions to get 1 cup cooked.

3. In a large bowl, combine baby arugula and warm barley, tossing until greens are slightly softened. Gently stir in beets, strawberries, and walnuts.

4. Divide the salad between two medium bowls. Drizzle the remaining olive oil, remaining lemon juice, and remaining balsamic vinegar equally between the two bowls.

5. Add a teaspoon of goat cheese to each bowl, breaking pieces off between two fingers to dot the salad.

6. Finally, add a few grinds of fresh black pepper over each salad to taste.

Substitution options: Try this with other baby greens that will wilt gently with a little warmth, such as baby spinach. Try other whole grains that keep their shape well in salads, such as wheatberry or farro.

Level-up: Excellent olive oil and balsamic vinegar will make all the difference in this salad. If you can't find aged balsamic, look for products marked balsamic glaze or balsamic reduction.

> **Nutrition:** 420 calories, 2810 mg omega-3s, 4 g saturated fat, 11 g protein, 36 g carbohydrates, 9 g fiber, 0 g added sugars, 530 mg potassium, 0.3 mg vitamin B6, 110 mcg folate, 0 mcg vitamin B12, 40 mg choline, 1570 mcg lutein

RED, WHITE, AND BLUE SALAD (WATERMELON BERRY SALAD)

Is it even summer if we're not eating watermelon? This one is perfect for patriotic celebrations and all the times in between. It's a simple treat for hot days made even simpler because there's no dressing to whisk. Instead, olive oil, lemon juice, and salt (in the form of feta) are added directly on top of the salad.

MIND foods: Leafy greens, berries, olive oil
Yield: 4 (1½-cup) servings | **Time:** 15 minutes

2 cups packed baby arugula
4 cups diced watermelon
1 cup blueberries
15–20 fresh mint leaves, hand torn
zest and juice of 1 large lemon

2 teaspoons sheep's milk feta
1 tablespoon olive oil
3–4 grinds freshly ground black
    pepper

1. To a large serving plate, lay a bed of arugula as the base layer. Top with watermelon, then sprinkle with blueberries.

2. Garnish with hand-torn mint leaves and lemon zest, aiming to distribute them evenly.

3. Gently crumble the feta over the salad as an additional garnish.

4. Finally drizzle lemon juice and olive oil over the salad and finish with freshly ground black pepper.

Notes: If a microplane isn't available, use a regular zester or simply slice the lemon peel with a knife, being careful not to pick up any of the bitter white pith and mince. The lemon zest can also be omitted and the salad will still be plenty lemony.

Substitution options: For people who love the briny flavor feta brings to this salad, try adding sliced olives to this salad.

Level-up: A good-quality olive oil and strong sheep's milk feta will make this salad sing. There aren't that many recipes in this book with cheese, so you know it's important. That said, I've made this salad without the feta and it's still great and super refreshing.

> **Nutrition:** 90 calories, 90 mg omega-3s, 1 g saturated fat, 2 g protein, 15 g carbohydrates, 2 g fiber, 0 g added sugars, 240 mg potassium, 0.1 mg vitamin B6, 30 mcg folate, 0 mcg vitamin B12, 10 mg choline, 810 mcg lutein

FARRO SALAD WITH CHOPPED HERBED CHICKEN

Just say no to boring salads with this vibrant salad featuring baby greens, tossed with warm farro, juicy strawberries, and crunchy cucumbers. Plant foods are the star, while chicken is an important but supporting cast member. Between the textures, flavors, and variety of ingredients, this salad offers everything you need for a deliciously balanced meal, plus an excellent source of protein, fiber, vitamin E, and vitamin B6, and a good source of iron, potassium, and choline.

MIND foods: Leafy greens, more vegetables, berries, nuts, whole grains, olive oil

Yield: 4 (large-salad) servings | **Time:** 10 minutes

4 cups lightly packed baby dark leafy greens, such as baby kale, baby spinach, or a mix

2½ cups cooked farro made with ½ teaspoon Diamond Crystal kosher salt (1 cup uncooked), ideally warm

15 medium strawberries, sliced

7-inch Korean cucumber, quartered lengthwise and chopped into ½-inch pieces

3 (5-inch) perilla leaves, rolled and cut into thin strips

1 cup chopped cooked chicken

¼ cup roughly chopped almonds

freshly ground black pepper, to taste

DRESSING INGREDIENTS

¼ cup olive oil

⅛ cup sherry vinegar

2 tablespoons fresh lemon juice

½ teaspoon Dijon mustard

¼ teaspoon garlic powder

¼ teaspoon ground ginger

¼ teaspoon honey

½ teaspoon Diamond Crystal kosher salt

1. In a small bowl, whisk together all the dressing ingredients.

2. In a large mixing bowl, combine the greens, cooked farro, strawberries, cucumber, perilla leaves, chicken, and dressing. Toss to combine and transfer to a serving bowl.

3. Garnish with almonds. Top with a few grinds of freshly ground black pepper to taste.

Notes: Korean perilla leaf is an aromatic herb related to mint and basil. It resembles shiso but has a unique flavor all its own. Find it at Korean markets. If you're unable to find it, use 15 to 20 fresh mint leaves. Korean cucumbers have a thin light-green mild-tasting skin, which can be left on or scored to keep half of it on. If you're unable to find it, use English, Kirby, or Persian cucumber.

Substitution options: To make this vegan, replace chicken with crispy tofu or black beans.

Nutrition: 400 calories, 190 mg omega-3s, 3 g saturated fat, 26 g protein, 34 g carbohydrates, 8 g fiber, 0 g added sugars, 700 mg potassium, 0.5 mg vitamin B6, 40 mcg folate, 0.2 mcg vitamin B12, 70 mg choline, 110 mcg lutein

POWER GREENS WITH CHICKEN AND SHERRY VINAIGRETTE

Dark green leafy vegetables are one of the best foods for brain health. This salad uses baby-sized leaves for their tender texture and less bitter taste. Plus, there's less prep because the leaves are already bite-sized. Lean poultry, beautiful strawberries, and earthy walnuts round out this salad, which is an excellent source of protein, vitamin E, potassium, and vitamin B6. It also provides a good source of fiber, iron, and choline.

MIND foods: Leafy greens, berries, nuts, lean poultry, olive oil, wine

Yield: 1 salad | **Time:** 20 minutes

2 cups baby dark leafy greens, such as baby kale, baby chard, baby spinach, or a combination
½ cup diced cooked chicken breast

½ cup quartered strawberries
2 teaspoons Dressing
2 tablespoons chopped walnuts

CHICKEN INGREDIENTS

1 pound skinless chicken breast, cut into ¾-inch cubes
½ teaspoon Diamond Crystal kosher salt

2 pinches of freshly ground black pepper
1 teaspoon Herbes de Provence
2 tablespoons olive oil
¼ cup sweet vermouth

DRESSING INGREDIENTS

2 tablespoons extra-virgin olive oil
1½ tablespoons balsamic vinegar

¼ teaspoon Diamond Crystal kosher salt

1. Season the chicken with salt, pepper, and Herbes de Provence.

2. Heat the olive oil in a medium nonstick pan over medium heat, about 2 minutes. Add the chicken in one layer and cook undisturbed, 2 minutes.

3. Flip the chicken and cover the pan for 2 minutes. Uncover, then drain oil. Add sweet vermouth, shaking in a circular motion occasionally, 2 more minutes. Turn heat off and rest the chicken, 3 minutes.

4. In a small bowl, whisk together all the dressing ingredients. Set aside.

5. In a large bowl, combine greens, ½ cup cooked chicken, and strawberries, and toss with 2–3 teaspoons of the dressing. Add to a bowl, top with walnuts, and enjoy.

Notes: You'll have leftover sherry vinaigrette and chopped chicken, both of which you can use in the Farro Salad with Chopped Herbed Chicken on page 187.

> **Nutrition:** 410 calories, 1490 mg omega-3s, 3 g saturated fat, 30 g protein, 13 g carbohydrates, 4 g fiber, 0 g added sugars, 930 mg potassium, 1 mg vitamin B6, 40 mcg folate, 0.2 mcg vitamin B12, 100 mg choline, 10 mcg lutein

KALE SALAD WITH JAMMY EGGS AND CRUNCHY CHICKPEAS

Hearty lacinato kale meets its match with a bold turmeric-Dijon dressing made with nutritional yeast ("Nooch"), yet the overall dish makes for a light and balanced meal complete with fiber-rich beans, jammy eggs, and peppery crisp radishes. A serving of this salad is rich in protein, fiber, vitamin E, vitamin B6, folate, vitamin B12, and choline. It's also a good source of calcium and iron.

MIND foods: Leafy greens, more vegetables, seafood, nuts, beans, olive oil
Yield: 2 (medium-salad) servings | **Time:** 1 hour 30 minutes

CRUNCHY CHICKPEAS

1 (15-ounce) can chickpeas, drained, rinsed

1½ tablespoons olive oil

½ teaspoon Diamond Crystal kosher salt

½ teaspoon freshly ground black pepper

½ teaspoon ground cumin

¼ teaspoon smoked paprika

SALAD

9 leaves lacinato kale, stems removed, cut into thin strips crosswise

¼ teaspoon Diamond Crystal kosher salt

2 medium round red radishes, trimmed, halved, and cut into ⅛-inch half-moons

2 tablespoons Nooch Sauce (page 192)

2 eggs

1. Drain and rinse the chickpeas, swirling them in a colander under streaming water until they stop foaming. Lay the chickpeas in one layer between two towels and gently roll them. Spend a few minutes removing skins that have come loose. Don't worry about doing them all.

2. Preheat the oven to 350°F for 15 minutes.

3. In a large bowl, wilt the kale by massaging it with ¼ teaspoon salt, 30 seconds. Add the radishes, then toss with the Nooch Sauce. Set aside.

4. In another large bowl, combine all the crunchy chickpea ingredients and toss to coat. Transfer to a medium rimmed sheet pan lined with a silicone mat, spreading them in one layer. Set the large bowl with remaining spice mix aside for later.

5. Roast the chickpeas for 45 minutes, opening the oven every 15 minutes to shake and rotate the pan. They are done when they have lost 30 to 50 percent of their original size, are crunchy, and are lightly browned but not dark. Watch them closely toward the end. The last 15 minutes may be split into 5-minute increments so that they don't overcook.

6. While the chickpeas are roasting, make the jammy eggs. Cover 2 eggs with cold water in a small pot with tight-fitting lid, bring the water to a boil, then turn off the heat. Cover the pot with the lid for 11 minutes. Prep an ice bath in a large bowl with ice and water. When cool enough to handle, peel the eggs and cut them in half lengthwise. Set aside.

7. When the chickpeas are done, transfer them back to the large bowl with remaining spice mix and swirl to coat. Add a teaspoon more oil if it seems dry. Transfer them back to the sheet pan to cool until ready to use.

8. To serve, divide the kale between two plates. To each plate, add two egg halves and ¼ cup of chickpeas. Let any extra chickpeas cool for at least 30 minutes before transferring to an airtight container and storing in a cool dry place for 4 to 5 days.

Notes: This meal can come together in under half an hour if the crunchy chickpeas and Nooch Sauce are made ahead of time. If you have them already made, you can sub in the Crunchy Spiced Chickpeas (page 181) here too.

Using a metal colander to swirl the chickpeas while rinsing them provides enough friction to help loosen the skins.

For jammier eggs, let them sit in hot water for 9 minutes instead of 11. For more well-done eggs, wait 12 minutes.

The crispy chickpeas will stay crispy for days but will taste best in the first days after roasting. For more snacking pleasure, the recipe can be doubled.

Level-up: Removing the skins, which hold some moisture, helps the chickpeas crisp up. If time and patience allow, remove all the skins. This is also a fun job for kitchen helpers (e.g., kids, friends, family).

NOOCH SAUCE

Yield: ¼ cup nooch sauce

1 clove garlic, roughly chopped
1½ fillets anchovy, from canned or jarred in oil
1 teaspoon Dijon mustard
¼ teaspoon ground turmeric

1 tablespoon nutritional yeast
¼ cup unsalted cashews
¼ cup fresh lemon juice
¼ cup avocado oil

1. Combine the garlic, anchovy, Dijon mustard, turmeric, nutritional yeast, and cashews in a mini food processor. Set to puree and pulse at 3-second intervals to combine. Stream in the lemon juice slowly to avoid it splashing out; repeat with the avocado oil until well blended.

> **Nutrition:** 430 calories, 240 mg omega-3s, 5 g saturated fat, 15 g protein, 28 g carbohydrates, 7 g fiber, 0 g added sugars, 270 mg potassium, 0.9 mg vitamin B6, 110 mcg folate, 1.1 mcg vitamin B12, 160 mg choline, 200 mcg lutein

CRISP GREENS & GRAPES SALAD

The crisp fresh greens and sweet red grapes come together with a simple vinaigrette in this salad. It tastes like a sweet spring day on a plate, and it is so good.

MIND foods: Leafy greens

Yield: 3 (large-salad) servings | **Time:** 15–20 minutes

2 tablespoons champagne vinegar
2 teaspoons avocado oil
¼ teaspoon Dijon mustard
1 teaspoon minced shallot, divided

2 pinches of Diamond Crystal kosher salt
2 hearts romaine, hand-torn into bite-sized pieces
20 small red grapes, halved

1. In a medium bowl, make the dressing by whisking together the vinegar, oil, mustard, ½ teaspoon of minced shallot, and salt. Set aside.

2. To a large serving platter, add the romaine, top with grapes, sprinkle on the remaining ½ teaspoon minced shallots, then drizzle with the dressing.

Substitution options: Good substitutes for champagne vinegar are prosecco vinegar and aged white wine vinegar. If your red grapes are particularly large, use 10 instead of 20 and quarter them.

SNAPS & BLUBS SALAD

Mother nature gives us so many naturally sweet flavors from fruits and vegetables alike. Sugar snap peas and sweet-tart blueberries are some of my favorite, which is why I have nicknames for them: snaps and blubs. I hope you become good friends with them, too. A large salad provides a good source of protein, iron, and folate.

MIND foods: More vegetables, berries, olive oil

Yield: 2 (large-salad) servings| **Time:** 15–20 minutes

2⅓ cups (1-inch) pieces sugar snap
   peas
½ heaping cup fresh blueberries
10 mint leaves, torn

DRESSING INGREDIENTS

2 tablespoons olive oil
1 tablespoon champagne vinegar
1 tablespoon minced shallot

1 teaspoon Dijon mustard
¼ teaspoon Diamond Crystal kosher
   salt

1.   Whisk all salad dressing ingredients together in a medium bowl, then set aside.

2.   Add the sugar snap peas and blueberries to the bowl of dressing and toss to coat. Transfer to a serving plate. Garnish with mint leaves.

SHAVED BRUSSELS SPROUTS, FIGS & FENNEL SALAD

This salad only gets better over time as the hearty yet delicate brussels sprouts and fennel soak up the dressing. Double the recipe for a crowd or make it ahead of time. It will look beautiful on a holiday table for a fresh take on brussels sprouts. A cup of this salad is an excellent source of fiber and provides protein, vitamin E, iron, potassium, vitamin B6, and folate.

MIND foods: Leafy greens, more vegetables, nuts, olive oil

Yield: 5 (1-cup) servings | **Time:** 50 minutes

4 cups trimmed and thinly sliced brussels sprouts

¼ cup sliced fennel bulb

7 dried mission figs, halved lengthwise and cut into thin strips, divided

2 seedless mandarin oranges, peeled and separated

½ heaping cup coarsely chopped walnuts, divided

DRESSING INGREDIENTS

4 tablespoons olive oil

2 tablespoons champagne vinegar

2 tablespoons minced shallot

2 teaspoons Dijon mustard

½ teaspoon Diamond Crystal kosher salt

1. Whisk together all the dressing ingredients in a small bowl, then set aside.

2. If your fennel has stalks and fronds, trim them so you are left with the white bulb. Using a Y-peeler, shave off any discolored sections. Cut the bulb in half lengthwise, then cut one half in half again. With a flat side down, trim the core out by slicing it out at an angle so it comes out as a triangular wedge. Thinly slice the remaining fennel lengthwise or crosswise—chef's choice. Transfer to the bowl with the brussels sprouts.

3. Pour ¼ cup of dressing over the brussels-fennel mixture. Reserve the remaining dressing to add more to taste, or for another use. Massage everything together for 1 minute, then let rest 30 minutes.

4. Cut the dried figs in half lengthwise. Then, flat side down, cut each half into thin slices. Repeat with remaining figs.

5. Add most of the figs, most of the walnuts, and all of the mandarin segments to the brussels-fennel mix, tossing to combine. Save a small amount of figs and walnuts for garnish.

6. Just before serving, garnish with remaining figs and walnuts.

Notes: The dressing can be made ahead and in a larger batch so you can use it for this salad and others, like the Snaps & Blubs Salad on page 194.

Dried figs and walnuts will both stay fresher longer if stored in the refrigerator. As an added bonus, refrigerated dried figs are easier to slice.

> **Nutrition:** 230 calories, 1190 mg omega-3s, 2 g saturated fat, 5 g protein, 24 g carbohydrates, 6 g fiber, 0 g added sugars, 500 mg potassium, 0.3 mg vitamin B6, 60 mcg folate, 0 mcg vitamin B12, 20 mg choline, 1200 mcg lutein

Soups

TURKEY CHILI

This quick and light yet hearty chili tastes better with every day that passes, and it freezes well too. Learn the basics of this recipe and you'll be able to riff on it with whatever vegetables you have on hand. A cup of this chili is an excellent source of protein, fiber, vitamin B6, folate, and vitamin B12. It also provides a good source of vitamin E, iron, potassium, and choline.

MIND foods: Leafy greens, more vegetables, beans, olive oil, lean poultry

Yield: 10 (1-cup) servings | **Time:** 35 minutes

5 medium cloves garlic, chopped and rested for 10–15 minutes	½ teaspoon dried cumin seeds
	¼ teaspoon ground cumin
2 tablespoons olive oil	¼ teaspoon dried oregano
1 small white onion, chopped	¼ teaspoon smoked paprika

¼ teaspoon ground coriander

½ teaspoon Diamond Crystal kosher salt

⅛ teaspoon freshly ground black pepper

½ teaspoon crushed red pepper flakes, plus more to garnish (optional)

1 pound lean ground turkey (93 percent lean or more)

1 (15-ounce) can red kidney beans, drained and rinsed

1 (15-ounce) can black beans, drained and rinsed

2½ cups thinly sliced green cabbage, to garnish

10 sprigs fresh flat-leaf parsley, leaves only, roughly chopped, to garnish

2 green onion stalks, sliced into rounds, to garnish

1. Mince the garlic and let it rest while prepping other ingredients. This gives it time to activate antioxidant and anti-inflammatory compounds such as allicin.

2. In a small bowl, combine and stir together all the herbs and spices.

3. Heat a 4.5-quart cast-iron pot over medium heat for 30 to 60 seconds before adding olive oil. Heat for another 1 to 2 minutes, or until tiny bubbles form on a wooden spatula held upright and pushed into the oil.

4. Add the chopped white onion and sauté for 1 minute. Add about half of the spice mix and stir continuously for 30 seconds, or until fragrant.

5. Add the ground turkey and sprinkle with remaining half of spice mix. Let it cook undisturbed for 2 to 3 minutes until browned, flip, and repeat, cooking turkey for 5 to 7 minutes total. Break up turkey into pieces and stir to coat pieces in spices.

6. Add the beans and tomatoes, stir, and bring to a simmer, stirring occasionally, about 5 minutes total.

7. Add the corn and bring the chili back to a simmer, about 2 minutes.

8. Turn the heat off, then stir in the vinegar and date paste.

9. Serve in individual bowls. Top each bowl with a ¼ cup of cabbage, a pinch each of parsley, green onion, and red pepper flakes, if using. Alternatively, set toppings on a table for self-service.

Notes: Tip: Give your canned goods a quick rinse and wipe-down. You don't know where they've been before they got to your kitchen.

Substitution options: For a soupier chili, add a cup of your broth of choice after the tomatoes. If you have leftover roasted vegetables, chop them up and replace 1 to 1½ cups of the corn. Cubes of roasted butternut squash would go great in this chili. To reduce spiciness, omit the red pepper flakes and replace with paprika. Or, for mild to medium smoky heat, replace the red chili flakes with 1 to 2 teaspoons gochugaru.

Level-up: Did you know you can make your own date paste at home with two simple ingredients? Check out my recipe on No-Bake Chewy Granola Balls on page 170.

Nutrition: 230 calories, 160 mg omega-3s, 2 g saturated fat, 15 g protein, 27 g carbohydrates, 7 g fiber, 0 g added sugars, 630 mg potassium, 0.4 mg vitamin B6, 80 mcg folate, 0.5 mcg vitamin B12, 60 mg choline, 430 mcg lutein

GREEN DREAM SOUP

Light yet flavorful with simple healthy flavors, the spiced chicken is the perfect complement to the vegetal soup. A serving of this soup is packed with protein and provides an excellent source of fiber, vitamin E, iron, potassium, vitamin B6, folate, and choline. It's also a good source of calcium and vitamin B12.

MIND foods: Leafy greens, more vegetables, beans, olive oil, lean poultry

Yield: 4 (1¼-cup soup and 3-ounce chicken) servings | **Time:** 35–40 minutes

12 ounces Basic Poached Chicken (page 222)
1 inch fresh ginger

3 tablespoons + 2 teaspoons olive oil, divided

3½ packed cup bite-sized cauliflower florets

2½ packed cups bite-sized broccoli florets

½ + ¼ teaspoon Diamond Crystal kosher salt, divided

2 cups chicken broth

4 cups baby kale, spinach, or chard

½ cup soft silken tofu

1 cup tightly packed fresh flat leaf parsley

½ teaspoon gochugaru (optional)

1. Rest the chicken at room temperature while the water comes to a boil. If the breasts are more than an inch thick, trim to ¾ to 1-inch thick.

2. In a medium pot with a tight-fitting lid, bring water to boil over high heat. There should be enough water to comfortably cover chicken breasts by at least a half-inch when in a single layer.

3. Add garlic and ginger to mini food processor and pulse for 3 to 5 seconds until minced. Set aside to rest for 15 minutes to let beneficial compounds develop. Prep and measure out other ingredients while it rests.

4. When the water is boiling, add the chicken in a single layer and bring the water back to a boil, then cover, turn heat off immediately, and remove the pot from the heat source. Keep covered to hold steam in, 20 minutes. A little longer is OK as this is a gentle cooking method.

5. Heat a large pot over medium-low heat, 30 seconds. Add 2 tablespoons of olive oil and heat, 1½ minutes.

6. Sauté the ginger and garlic, 30 seconds or until fragrant. Don't let the garlic burn.

7. Add the cauliflower, broccoli, and ½ teaspoons salt and stir to coat, 1 minute.

8. Pour in the chicken broth, increase heat to high, and bring to a boil. Lower heat to a steady simmer, cover, and cook, 8 minutes more.

9. Remove from heat. Using an immersion blender, blend until smooth. Ensure blades are fully immersed in liquid. Move the blender to different spots until everything is blended and the blender easily makes contact with the bottom of the pot.

10. Add the baby greens and repeat. Add the tofu and repeat. Add the parsley and repeat. When there is enough liquid to do so, holding the immersion blender at a slight angle will allow better circulation through its blades.

11. Toss Poached Chicken with 2 teaspoons olive oil, gochugaru, if using, and ¼ teaspoon salt.

12. To serve, divide the soup into 4 bowls and top each with even amounts of shredded chicken.

Substitution options: To make this completely plant based, omit the chicken and replace the chicken broth with vegetable broth.

> **Nutrition:** 350 calories, 350 mg omega-3s, 3 g saturated fat, 36 g protein, 13 g carbohydrates, 6 g fiber, 0 g added sugars, 1130 mg potassium, 1 mg vitamin B6, 90 mcg folate, 0.3 mcg vitamin B12, 110 mg choline, 3250 mcg lutein

CAULIFLOWER SOUP

With the comforting consistency of potato soup, this cauliflower soup includes a few surprising gifts from the sea to help boost flavor while increasing your weekly seafood intake. The serving size on this one is smaller because it packs so much flavor. Each Half cup provides a good source of protein, vitamin E, and iron.

MIND foods: More vegetables, seafood, whole grains, olive oil

Yield: 4 (½-cup) servings | **Time:** 22 minutes

6–8 cups cauliflower florets
3 tablespoons plus 2 teaspoons olive oil, divided
1 anchovy fillet, from tinned in oil

1 teaspoon doenjang
2 cloves garlic, minced
1½ cups low-sodium chicken broth
6 (⅓-inch) slices multigrain baguette

1 (6.5-ounce) can chopped clams in clam juice

¼ teaspoon Diamond Crystal kosher salt, divided, plus more to taste

freshly ground black pepper, to taste

1 sprig fresh flat-leaf parsley, leaves only, chopped

1. In a large food processor, pulse the cauliflower until it resembles rice, 1½ minutes.

2. In a medium pot, heat 3 tablespoons of olive oil on medium-low heat, 2 minutes. Add the anchovy and doenjang, mash both into oil, and stir, 60 seconds. Add garlic and stir, 60 seconds or until fragrant.

3. Add the broth, increasing the heat to bring broth to a boil. Add the cauliflower and reduce heat to a simmer, 7 minutes.

4. While the cauliflower heats, make the garlic toast. Add 2 teaspoons of olive oil to a medium nonstick pan over medium heat, 2 minutes. Add the baguette slices and toast for 2 minutes, or until lightly browned, flip, and repeat for 2 minutes. Transfer to a plate, rub one side of toast with raw garlic, and sprinkle with salt. Set aside.

5. Using an immersion blender, blend the soup until smooth, moving the blender around the pot, 5 minutes.

6. Stir in the chopped clams and clam juice until warmed through, 1 minute. Taste and season with salt if needed.

7. To serve, divide the soup into two bowls. Add a few grinds of freshly ground black pepper and fresh parsley. Serve with 3 garlic toasts per serving.

Notes: Doenjang is a funkier Korean cousin to miso that is available at Korean markets, some Asian markets, or online. If it's unavailable, substitute with miso or soy sauce.

Nutrition: 200 calories, 120 g omega-3s, 2 g saturated fat, 8 g protein, 11 g carbohydrates, 2 g fiber, 0 g added sugars, 270 mg potassium, 0.05 mg vitamin B6, 0 mcg folate, 0.1 mcg vitamin B12, 0 mg choline, 10 mcg lutein

Sides

ROASTED BROCCOLI WITH NOOCH SAUCE

Roasting the broccoli low and slow makes this super craveable—with or without the sauce, but the sauce in this recipe takes the flavor up a notch.

MIND foods: More vegetables, nuts, seafood, nuts, olive oil

Yield: 5 (½-cup) servings | **Time:** 55 minutes

BROCCOLI

5 cups broccoli florets

3 tablespoons olive oil

¼ teaspoon Diamond Crystal kosher salt

¼ teaspoon freshly ground black pepper

2 tablespoons Nooch Sauce (page 192)

1½ tablespoons chopped almonds

1. Preheat the oven to 325°F for 15 minutes.

2. In a large bowl, combine the broccoli with the olive oil, salt, and pepper, making sure to coat all pieces until they are shiny and look wet. Transfer to a rack fitted into a large rimmed sheet pan.

3. Roast the broccoli for 20 minutes, shake and rotate the pan, and return to the oven for 20 more minutes. Taste and check for doneness. Broccoli should be about half its original size when cooked. Some browned tips are OK, but you don't want to burn the broccoli. Return to the oven for another 5 minutes if needed.

4. Let broccoli cool for 5 to 10 minutes. Toss with 2 tablespoons of Nooch Sauce just before serving.

5. Transfer to a serving dish and garnish with chopped almonds. Optional: if you'd like to brighten the dish, squeeze the juice of a quarter-lemon over the broccoli just before eating.

Notes: Nooch sauce can also be used in the Kale Salad with Jammy Eggs and Crunchy Chickpeas (page 190).

WARM FONIO AND ASPARAGUS PILAF WITH RED GRAPES

If you haven't heard of fonio, be ready to meet your new favorite quick-cooking whole grain. Fonio is an ancient West African whole grain that cooks up in 5 minutes. It's also naturally gluten-free in case you or someone in your household needs gluten-free options. The sweet pops of flavor from the red grapes wonderfully balance out the grassy vegetal asparagus.

MIND foods: More vegetables, whole grains, olive oil

Yield: 5 (¾-cup) servings | **Time:** 15–20 minutes

1 cup chopped asparagus spears
3 teaspoons olive oil, divided
¼ teaspoon Diamond Crystal kosher salt, divided
2 pinches of freshly ground black pepper

½ cup fonio
1 cup low-sodium chicken broth
1½ cups halved small red grapes
6–10 fresh mint leaves, torn

1. Trim the asparagus, holding the stem and bending the spear away from it until it snaps. Cut into 1-inch pieces on the diagonal.

2. In a medium pot with a tight-fitting lid, heat 1 teaspoon of olive oil over medium heat, 1 minute. Add the asparagus, a pinch of salt, and black pepper, stirring occasionally, 3 minutes.

3. Add the fonio, remaining 2 teaspoons of olive oil, and remaining salt, then stir to coat. Add the broth and bring to a boil. Turn heat off, cover with lid, and wait 5 minutes. Fluff with a fork.

4. Gently stir the grapes into the finished fonio-asparagus mixture. Transfer to a serving platter. Garnish with torn mint leaves.

Notes: Fonio is available in grocery stores and online.

Substitution options: This would also work well with snow peas, sugar snap peas, zucchini, summer squash, or bell peppers in place of the asparagus. If you can't find fonio, whole wheat cous cous is a great substitute, but keep in mind that it will no longer be gluten-free.

> **Nutrition:** 150 calories, 30 mg omega-3s, 1 g saturated fat, 3 g protein, 28 g carbohydrates, 2 g fiber, 0 g added sugars, 210 mg potassium, 0.1 mg vitamin B6, 20 mcg folate, 0.1 mcg vitamin B12, 10 mg choline, 240 mcg lutein

CITRUS SPICED CARROTS

These are so good, I've been known to eat a whole batch while still standing in the kitchen. Tangy lemon and orange notes balance with warm spices in this delicious Moroccan-inspired carrot side dish. That said, gochugaru is a uniquely Korean ingredient that falls outside spices commonly used in Moroccan cuisine, yet lends some of the same mild smoky heat that might otherwise come from white pepper or red chili peppers.

MIND foods: More vegetables, olive oil

Yield: 4 (½-cup) servings | **Time:** 20 minutes

CARROTS

1 pound carrots, peeled and trimmed
3 tablespoons orange juice
1 tablespoon Spice Blend
1½ tablespoons olive oil

1 tablespoon fresh lemon juice
2 pinches Diamond Crystal kosher salt
5–10 large fresh mint leaves, torn

SPICE BLEND

1 tablespoon ground coriander
1 tablespoon ground cumin
1 tablespoon gochugaru

1 tablespoon garlic powder
1 tablespoon smoked paprika
1 tablespoon ground turmeric

1. Combine all the ingredients for the spice blend. You will have extra, which you can use for the Juicy Chicken Shawarma Pita Pockets (page 226).

2. Using a food processor with a slicing blade, process the carrots into ⅛-inch rounds. Place in a large microwave-safe bowl with orange juice and microwave, covered, 4 minutes. Keep covered until ready to use.

3. Heat a large pan over medium heat, 30 seconds.

4. Toast 1 tablespoon of spice blend in the pan, stirring until fragrant and darker in color, 1 minute.

5. Add olive oil and swirl, then stir in the orange juice, 30 seconds.

6. Add lemon juice and stir continuously as it bubbles, 30 seconds.

7. Add the sliced carrots and the orange juice they were steamed in to the pan. Stir to coat in spices. Season with salt. Cook, stirring occasionally, 3 minutes. Liquid will have reduced and become saucy. Carrots should be cooked through and semisoft but not mushy. Optional: cook for an additional couple minutes for softer carrots, but stop if the pan gets dry and spices stick to the bottom of the pan.

8. Transfer carrots to a serving platter and garnish with freshly torn mint leaves.

Notes: If a food processor with slicing blade is not available, use a mandoline or chef's knife and add 3 to 5 minutes to the prep time.

Note that lemons give varying levels of juice. You might get away with using half a lemon or may need most of 1 lemon to get to the tablespoon lemon juice used in this recipe. Plan accordingly.

Nutrition: 130 calories, 40 mg omega-3s, 1 g saturated fat, 2 g protein, 24 g carbohydrates, 7 g fiber, 0 g added sugars, 770 mg potassium, 0.3 mg vitamin B6, 50 mcg folate, 0 mcg vitamin B12, 20 mg choline, 620 mcg lutein

GARLIC-GINGER BABY BOK CHOY

I wanted to make this with pea shoots, which are so, so good and relatively high in protein for a leafy green, but they're not always easy to find, so I opted for some lovely baby bok choy, which is just as delicious. Super flavorful and nutritious, this side dish can be on the table in under 15 minutes.

MIND foods: Leafy greens, olive oil

Yield: 2 (½-cup) servings | **Time:** 10–15 minutes

2 heads baby bok choy

1 tablespoon olive oil

2 pinches Diamond Crystal kosher salt, divided

3 medium cloves garlic, minced

¼-inch fresh ginger, minced

1 tablespoon unsweetened rice wine

1. Wash the baby bok choy in a large bowl of cold water. Pull the leaves off by applying gentle outward pressure with your thumb from the inside base of each leaf, near the stem. Transfer to another bowl, rinse debris from first bowl and repeat if necessary, until water is clear. Set over a colander to dry.

2. Heat a 10-inch nonstick pan over medium heat, 30 seconds. Add the olive oil and heat, 1½ minutes. Add the baby bok choy leaves and toss with kitchen tongs to coat, until the leaves are slightly wilted, 1 minute.

3. Season the baby bok choy with a pinch of salt and continue to cook, gently mixing with the kitchen tongs occasionally, 2 more minutes.

4. Add the garlic and ginger, tossing with tongs continuously, 30 seconds.

5. Pour the rice wine over the pan and continue to toss with tongs, 1 minute. Remove from the heat and transfer to a serving plate. Season with the remaining pinch of salt. Enjoy.

Substitution options: This would be amazing with pea shoots, as mentioned above. This method would also work wonders on snow peas.

BLACK BEAN PICO DE GALLO

I grew up in southern California eating pico de gallo, aka salsa fresca, with delicious Mexican food. I love the fresh flavors that are distinct yet well-married components in this kind of salsa. Tomatoes are usually the main attraction, but black beans are the star of this dish. Enjoy it as a side dish, dip, on top of flaky white fish, or wrapped in a soft warm corn tortilla.

MIND foods: More vegetables, beans, olive oil

Yield: 13 (½-cup) servings | **Time:** 45 minutes

DRESSING INGREDIENTS

zest from 2 limes
2 tablespoons lime juice
¼ cup olive oil
2 tablespoons red wine vinegar
1 clove garlic

2 pinches of crushed red pepper
   flakes
½ teaspoon ground cumin
½ teaspoon Diamond Crystal kosher
   salt
½ teaspoon freshly ground black
   pepper

SALSA INGREDIENTS

2 (15-ounce) cans black beans, drained
   and rinsed
1½ cups Roma tomatoes, deseeded
   and diced
1½ cups frozen sweet corn kernels
1 small red onion, chopped

1 medium jalapeño, trimmed,
   deseeded, and chopped
1 medium avocado, diced
½ cup packed cilantro, chopped
½ teaspoon Diamond Crystal kosher
   salt (optional)

1. Combine all the dressing ingredients in a personal inverted blender and blend until the garlic is well incorporated. Set aside.

2. In a large bowl, layer the black beans, tomatoes, corn, red onion, jalapeno, avocado, and cilantro.

3. Pour the dressing over the salad and use a wide spoon such as a serving spoon or wooden kitchen spoon to gently bring the black beans from the bottom up to the top. Rotate the bowl a quarter of a turn and repeat until the salsa is well combined. Taste and season with ½ teaspoon salt, if needed. Stir with the same method to distribute salt throughout.

4. Enjoy immediately or let rest and marinate for at least an hour to allow flavors to develop. Refrigerate in an airtight container for up to 4 days.

Notes: This one is great for a crowd. It doesn't freeze well, so if you don't think you'll be able to finish it, cut the recipe in half.

This dish is best when all the elements are knife-cut, but as a timesaver, a mini-food processor can be used on the onion, after cutting it in quarters, and the jalapeño, after cutting it in two pieces. Simply pulse on the chop setting in 1-second increments until they are chopped but not soupy, 5 to 10 pulses. This is not recommended for the tomatoes, cilantro, or avocado, as they are too delicate.

Substitution options: If spicy isn't your thing, omit the jalapeño and crushed red pepper flakes. For a milder heat, replace the red pepper flakes with half as much gochugaru.

Nutrition: 140 calories, 120 mg omega-3s, 1 g saturated fat, 4 g protein, 18 g carbohydrates, 6 g fiber, 0 g added sugars, 330 mg potassium, 0.2 mg vitamin B6, 80 mcg folate, 0 mcg vitamin B12, 20 mg choline, 240 mcg lutein

SWEET POTATO PANCAKES

Sweet potato pancakes might sound like breakfast—and they absolutely can be—but there's no rule that pancakes have to be breakfast. Snack on one of these any time of day for a sweet and savory way to get some vitamin A.

MIND foods: More vegetables, whole grains, olive oil
Yield: 9 (1-pancake) servings | **Time:** 40 minutes

1 pound sweet potatoes, peeled, quartered lengthwise
1 tablespoon whole wheat flour
2 eggs
1 tablespoon dried parsley
1 tablespoon dried thyme
1 teaspoon garlic powder
½ teaspoon + pinch of Diamond Crystal kosher salt, divided
½ teaspoon freshly ground black pepper
2 tablespoons + 1 teaspoon olive oil, divided

1. In a food processor with a grating blade, shred the sweet potatoes.

2. In a large bowl, microwave the shredded potatoes, covered, 3 minutes. Stir, then re-cover and microwave for another 3 minutes. Taste. Shreds should be softened and nearly fully cooked but not mushy. If needed, stir and microwave, covered, for another minute.

3. Lightly dust the sweet potatoes with the flour, a little at a time, tossing then dusting a few times to evenly incorporate the flour.

4. Whisk the eggs in a small bowl with the parsley, thyme, garlic powder, ½ teaspoon of salt, and pepper. Add to the large bowl with the sweet potatoes and gently stir to coat the potatoes thoroughly with egg mixture.

5. Heat a 10-inch nonstick pan over medium to medium-low heat, 30 seconds. Add 1 tablespoon of olive oil and heat for 1½ minutes.

6. Pack sweet potatoes into a ¼ cup scoop before transferring to the pan. Press down with the back of the scoop to flatten pancakes to ¼-inch or less. Working in batches of 3 to 4 pancakes, cook for 4 minutes, flip, then cook for an additional 3 minutes or until golden-brown. Add 2 teaspoons of oil before each batch. Transfer cooked pancakes to a wire rack, sprinkle with salt.

7. These pancakes pair nicely with plain yogurt or Green Sauce (page 163).

Notes: If you don't have a food processor with a grating plate, use the largest shredding holes on a box grater or handheld grater. Also, keep in mind that the first batch always takes a little longer to cook.

> **Nutrition:** 100 calories, 40 mg omega-3s, 1 g saturated fat, 2 g protein, 12 g carbohydrates, 2 g fiber, 0 g added sugars, 200 mg potassium, 0.1 mg vitamin B6, 12 mcg folate, 0.1 mcg vitamin B12, 40 mg choline, 50 mcg lutein

GARDEN PIE

There's shepherd's pie (made with lamb), cottage pie (made with beef), and now, garden pie (made with veggies), a hearty comforting dish topped with bright-orange sweet potatoes, signaling this isn't your average "meat" pie. Make it once and it will feed you for days with plenty of plant protein, omega-3s, and antioxidants. A serving is an excellent source of protein, fiber, iron, vitamin B6, and folate and a good source of vitamin E, potassium, and choline.

MIND foods: More vegetables, nuts, beans, whole grains, olive oil

Yield: 6 (1-cup) servings | **Time:** 1 hour

1½ cups walnut halves or pieces

1 (15-ounce) can black beans, drained, rinsed, divided

3 tablespoons + ½ teaspoon olive oil, divided

1 cup chopped red onion

1 tablespoon dried parsley

2 teaspoons dried thyme

1 teaspoon dried rosemary

3 pinches + ½ teaspoon Diamond Crystal kosher salt, divided

½ teaspoon freshly ground black pepper

2 cloves garlic, minced

1½ teaspoons doenjang paste

2 teaspoons apple cider vinegar

2 tablespoons whole wheat flour

2 tablespoons tomato paste

1 cup low-sodium chicken broth

1½ cups fresh or frozen sweet corn kernels

½ cup fresh or frozen peas

1 pound sweet potatoes, peeled

2 eggs

3 sprigs fresh flat leaf parsley, leaves only, chopped, to garnish (optional)

1. Combine the walnuts with half the black beans in a mini food processor set to chop. Pulse until coarsely chopped, 10 to 20 seconds.

2. Heat a large heavy-bottomed pot, such as a 2.5-quart cast-iron pot, over medium heat, 30 seconds. Add 2 tablespoons of olive oil and heat, 1½ minutes.

3. Add the chopped red onion, season with a pinch of salt, and stir occasionally, 3 to 5 minutes.

4. Add the walnut-black bean mixture and the remaining half of black beans, and mix together with the parsley, thyme, rosemary, ½ teaspoon salt, and pepper.

5. In a small bowl, whisk together the garlic paste, doenjang, and apple cider vinegar before mixing into the pot, 1 minute.

6. Dust the flour over the mixture and gently incorporate.

7. Make room in the pot to add ½ teaspoon olive oil and the tomato paste so it touches the bottom of the pot. Let it caramelize for 3 to 5 minutes. When it becomes a darker red, mix it into the larger mixture.

8. Preheat the oven to 400°F.

9. Pour the broth and frozen vegetables into the pot. Mix together, bring to a boil then lower heat to a simmer, stirring occasionally, 5 minutes.

10. In a food processor with a grating blade, shred the sweet potatoes. Microwave shredded potatoes in a large covered microwave-safe bowl for 3 minutes. Stir, then repeat to microwave, covered, for another 3 minutes. Taste. Shreds should be softened and nearly fully cooked but not mushy. If needed, stir and microwave for another minute.

11. Whisk the eggs in a small bowl with 1 tablespoon of olive oil and ⅛ teaspoon salt before pouring it over shredded sweet potatoes. Gently stir to coat potatoes thoroughly with egg mixture.

12. Transfer the walnut-bean "meat" mixture into an 8 x 11-inch baking dish. Top with the sweet potato mixture. Bake in oven for 10 minutes, rotate, bake for another 10, rotate, and if needed, bake for another 5 to 10 minutes. The tops of the sweet potato should be cooked but not singed.

13. Cool for 10 minutes. Garnish with fresh parsley, if using, and enjoy. This dish pairs nicely with a dollop of Green Sauce (page 163).

Notes: If you don't have a food processor with a grating plate, use the largest shredding holes on a box grater or handheld grater.

Substitution options: You can use any onion you have on hand. If doenjang is unavailable, use 1 tablespoon Worcestershire sauce in place of doenjang and apple cider vinegar.

> **Nutrition:** 460 calories, 2440 mg omega-3s, 3 g saturated fat, 14 g protein, 47 g carbohydrates, 11 g fiber, 0 g added sugars, 830 mg potassium, 0.5 mg vitamin B6, 130 mcg folate, 0.2 mcg vitamin B12, 90 mg choline, 800 mcg lutein

CHANA MASALA

This aromatic chickpea-based tomato stew offers a pleasant lingering heat you can feel but is not overwhelming. Still, if you prefer, you can cut the gochugaru in half or omit. It may look done after 10 minutes of simmering, but it's the next 10 minutes when something magical happens as the tomatoes caramelize a bit to create a richer flavor. This dish is inspired by the many bowls of chana masala I ate in the East Village of NYC in my twenties. A serving is rich in fiber and a good source of protein, vitamin D, vitamin E, iron, potassium, and folate.

MIND foods: More vegetables, beans, olive oil

Yield: 4 (1-cup) servings | **Time:** 45 minutes

1 medium yellow or white onion
1 inch fresh ginger
2 teaspoons gochugaru
1 teaspoon ground garam masala
1 teaspoon ground turmeric
1 teaspoon ground cumin

1 cinnamon stick
3 tablespoons olive oil
2 teaspoons cumin seeds
1 (28-ounce) can fire-roasted diced tomatoes, very-low sodium
1 clove garlic, minced

1 (15-ounce) can chickpeas, drained and rinsed

2 tablespoons fresh lime juice

¼ cup plain yogurt

1¼ teaspoons Diamond Crystal kosher salt

1. Peel, trim, and quarter the onion. Add the onion and ginger to a mini food processor. Set to puree and pulse until the onion and garlic are minced. Transfer to a prep bowl.

2. In a small prep bowl, combine the gochugaru, garam masala, turmeric, ground cumin, and cinnamon stick.

3. Heat a high-walled 10-inch skillet over medium heat, 30 seconds. Add olive oil and heat, 1½ minutes.

4. Add the cumin seeds and stir continuously, 30 seconds.

5. Add cinnamon stick-spice mixture and stir continuously, 1 minute.

6. Stir in minced onion-ginger mixture, stirring occasionally, 2 minutes.

7. Add tomatoes and cook, 2 minutes.

8. Add minced garlic and cook for 1 more minute.

9. Stir in chickpeas, lime juice, yogurt, and salt. Bring back to a strong simmer and cook for 20 minutes more. Five minutes in, use a potato masher to press down to the bottom of the pan 4 to 6 times to smash some—but not all—of the chickpeas. By the end, the stew will thicken and the tomatoes will have reduced, concentrating their sweetness. Serve with whole wheat naan or brown basmati rice, with a side of leafy greens.

Nutrition: 260 calories, 110 mg omega-3s, 2 g saturated fat, 8 g protein, 33 g carbohydrates, 8 g fiber, 0 g added sugars, 680 mg potassium, 0.1 mg vitamin B6, 40 mcg folate, 0.1 mcg vitamin B12, 30 mg choline, 20 mcg lutein

BIBIM GUKSU (BUCKWHEAT NOODLE BOWL)

You may have heard of bibimbap, a sizzling hot Korean mixed rice dish with vegetables, sometimes meat and/or an egg, and a savory sauce to bring it all together. This is bibim (mixed) guksu (noodles), a lighter cousin to bibimbap that is enjoyed cool or at room temperature, so it's perfect for hot days or anytime you want a fresh, balanced one-bowl meal. This bowl is rich in protein, fiber, and iron and provides a good source of calcium, potassium, vitamin B6, and folate.

MIND foods: Leafy greens, more vegetables, whole grains, olive oil

Yield: 1 bowl | **Time:** 15–20 minutes

1¼ inches medium Korean cucumber

1½ inches medium carrot

3.2-ounce bundle thin buckwheat noodles (look for under 120 mg sodium/serving)

¼ cup packed sliced Napa cabbage kimchi

1 teaspoon sesame oil

½ teaspoon olive oil

1 tablespoon apple cider vinegar

2 pinches teaspoon garlic powder

2 pinches teaspoon ground ginger

1 pinch of teaspoon Diamond Crystal kosher salt

1 teaspoon gochujang (optional)

1 cup packed spring mix baby greens

1. In a medium pot on high heat, boil 5 cups of water.

2. While the water is coming to a boil, cut the cucumber on a long diagonal into ⅛-inch oblong coins, then lay them flat to cut into ⅛-inch strips. Repeat with the carrot.

3. When the water comes to a boil, add the buckwheat noodles, stirring occasionally, 6 minutes.

4. While the noodles are cooking, make the dressing by stirring together the sesame oil, olive oil, apple cider vinegar, garlic powder, ground ginger, salt, and gochujang (if using) in a small bowl.

5. Use tongs to transfer noodles immediately to a large fine-mesh strainer set over a large bowl to catch dripping water. Move to the sink and rinse under running cold water, mixing occasionally until the noodles are cool to the touch.

6. Wipe out the large bowl used to catch dripping water from the buckwheat noodles. Combine all ingredients in the bowl and toss to coat with dressing. Transfer to a serving bowl and enjoy.

Notes: The gochujang provides a pleasant heat and subtle sweetness to the final dish, but if you are sensitive to spice, you may reduce the amount or omit.

For presentation, you have the option to place the spring mix greens at the bottom of a wide bowl. Top with noodles. Add kimchi, carrot, and cucumbers in separate sections on top of the noodles. Drizzle sauce on top.

Substitution options: If Korean cucumbers are unavailable, use any small-seed cucumber, including Kirby, Persian, or English cucumbers. To make this an even more substantial dish, you may top it with a jammy egg, poached chicken, or the salmon from the Doenjang Salmon Lettuce Wraps on page 215.

Nutrition: 460 calories, 70 mg omega-3s, 2 g saturated fat, 16 g protein, 77 g carbohydrates, 9 g fiber, 1 g added sugars, 560 mg potassium, 0.2 mg vitamin B6, 60 mcg folate, 0 mcg vitamin B12, 10 mg choline, 140 mcg lutein

DOENJANG SALMON LETTUCE WRAPS

These lettuce wraps have just the right balance of super-flavorful salmon, comforting warm rice, and fresh veggies. Korean food treats protein foods like condiments, which is why they're often very flavorful. This is balanced out by larger portions of whole grains and vegetables. Give this balance a try with these lettuce wraps. Each serving is protein rich and an excellent source of vitamin D, vitamin E, vitamin B6, folate, vitamin B12, and omega-3s. It also provides iron, potassium, and choline.

MIND foods: Leafy greens, more vegetables, seafood, whole grains, olive oil
Yield: 4 (½-cup) servings of flaked salmon plus lettuce wrap accompaniments |
Time: 18 minutes

1 tablespoon olive oil   1 pound frozen salmon fillets

2 tablespoons + 1 teaspoon rice wine, divided
2 teaspoons doenjang
2 teaspoons Date Paste (page 171)
1 teaspoon low-sodium soy sauce
1 teaspoon mirin
¼ teaspoon Diamond Crystal kosher salt
1 head butter lettuce or romaine
2 cups of cooked brown rice or whole grain medley
2 red radishes, cut into thin strips
½ cup shredded kimchi

1. If rice is not already made, cook rice according to package instructions or in a rice cooker.

2. Heat a large pan with a tight-fitting lid on medium-high, 30 seconds. Add olive oil and heat, 2 minutes. Add frozen salmon, skin side down (if it's skinless, you will still place it flat side down, where the skin would have been). Cook undisturbed, 3 minutes.

3. Flip, drizzle with 2 tablespoons rice wine, lower heat to medium, cover and cook undisturbed, 6 minutes.

4. Meanwhile, make the sauce by mixing the doenjang, date paste, soy sauce, mirin, 1 tsp of rice wine, and salt together in a small bowl until combined.

5. Separate the butter lettuce (or romaine) into individual leaves.

6. Quarter radishes and thinly slice.

7. When fish is done, uncover and add 2 tablespoons of sauce. With gentle pressure from a wooden kitchen spoon or spatula, break the salmon into flakes and mix with the sauce, 2 minutes or until all flakes of salmon are opaque. Fully cooked salmon should give way easily; if it doesn't, let it keep cooking undisturbed until it turns opaque.

8. Serve family style with lettuce, rice, salmon, radishes, and kimchi, if using, on the table for people to serve themselves. Each lettuce cup can have a spoonful of rice, a small spoonful of salmon, and a sprinkling of radishes and kimchi.

Notes: If you prefer not to eat the salmon skin, simply pick it out; however, it's where the highest concentration of omega-3s are.

If you are cooking salmon filets from fresh or thawed, leave it at room temperature for 10 to 15 minutes, then cook skin side down for about 6 minutes or until ¾ of the side of the fish looks opaque. Flip and cook for 1 to 2 more minutes, or until a quick read thermometer reads 145°F.

If you are cooking skinless salmon filets from fresh or thawed, cook about 5 minutes on one side or until about half the side of the fish looks opaque, flip then cook 4 minutes on the other side, or until a quick read thermometer reads 145°F.

Nutrition: 410 calories, 3090 mg omega-3s, 3 g saturated fat, 26 g protein, 32 g carbohydrates, 2 g fiber, 0 g added sugars, 870 mg potassium, 1.2 mg vitamin B6, 80 mcg folate, 3.5 mcg vitamin B12, 90 mg choline, 20 mcg lutein

FISH TACOS

Fish tacos are a fun family-style meal. This recipe uses a mild-tasting white fish, making it a good intro to seafood for kids and adults alike. A serving is high in protein, iron, and vitamin B12, and a good source of fiber, vitamin E, calcium, potassium, vitamin B6, and choline.

MIND foods: Leafy greens, seafood, whole grains, olive oil

Yield: 5 (2-taco) servings | **Time:** 30–35 minutes

1 pound Alaskan cod or other white fish
1 teaspoon smoked ground paprika
½ teaspoon ground cumin
1½ teaspoons gochugaru, divided
1 teaspoon Diamond Crystal kosher salt, divided
½ cup plain nonfat plain yogurt

2 tablespoons plus 1 teaspoon olive oil, divided
3 limes, divided
10 lacinato kale leaves, destemmed and sliced in thin strips
10 stalks cilantro, roughly chopped
10 (5½-inch) soft corn tortillas

1. Pat the fish dry and season it with the paprika, cumin, 1 teaspoon of gochugaru, and ½ teaspoon of salt.

2. Make the yogurt sauce by mixing together the yogurt, juice from 2 limes, 1 teaspoon of olive oil, ¼ teaspoon of salt, and ½ teaspoon of gochugaru.

3. Massage the kale with ¼ teaspoon salt, 30 seconds, then rest for 15 minutes. Then massage with ¼ cup of yogurt sauce and set aside.

4. Heat a 10-inch pan over medium heat, 30 seconds. Add 2 tablespoons of olive oil and heat, 1½ minutes. Add the cod, skin (or flat) side down and cook undisturbed, 3 to 5 minutes. Flip and cook for another 2 to 3 minutes or until fish flakes easily with a little downward angled pressure and all fish is opaque and 145°F. Turn off the heat and flake the remaining fish.

5. Wash, dry, and roughly chop the cilantro. Hold the lime on a long edge and cut a piece off the left and the right, away from the core. These are full lime cheeks. Flip the lime onto a flat edge and cut the other two sides. These are half cheeks. Cutting the lime this way make it easy to squeeze its juice.

6. Serve family style, using communal serving bowls for each of the following: tortillas, flaked cod, dressed kale slaw, chopped cilantro, extra yogurt sauce, and lime cheeks. The sauce can go on top of the taco or on the tortilla to help the fish stay in place. Top with cod, slaw, and cilantro. Top with squeeze of fresh lime juice.

Notes: To make this meal come together even quicker, the kale slaw can be made ahead of time and will taste all the better for having more time with the dressing.

Substitution options: Use any kind of seafood you like! Try other white fish, salmon, or even shellfish like shrimp. Add some sliced avocado to make the tacos more substantial.

Nutrition: 260 calories, 190 mg omega-3s, 1 g saturated fat, 21 g protein, 32 g carbohydrates, 4 g fiber, 0 g added sugars, 670 mg potassium, 0.2 mg vitamin B6, 16 mcg folate, 2.3 mcg vitamin B12, 80 mg choline, 120 mcg lutein

BASIC FISH FILLET COOKED FROM FROZEN, TWO WAYS

This basic recipe is for anyone who's ever worried about fish going bad before you have a chance to cook it (myself included!). Don't let that stop you from enjoying the benefits of eating fish. It cooks so quickly, it can easily be cooked from frozen. In fact, fish is often flash frozen on the seas at peak quality anyway.

MIND foods: Seafood, olive oil

Yield: 2 (4½-ounce) servings | **Time:** 15 minutes or less

PAN SEARING

2 (6-ounce, 1-inch-thick) fish fillets
3 teaspoons olive oil, divided

1. Pat fish dry with paper towels.

2. Heat a cast-iron nonstick pan over medium heat, 30 seconds. Add 2 teaspoons of olive oil to the pan and let heat, 1½ minutes.

3. Add fish fillet, skin (or flat) side down, cooking undisturbed for 4 minutes. Drizzle 1 teaspoon of olive oil over the top of the fillet as it cooks.

4. Flip the fillet. Sprinkle with salt, herbs, and spices as desired.

5. Cover and cook for 6 minutes more or until an instant-read thermometer inserted into the thickest part of the fish reads 145°F.

6. Fish will be opaque and flake easily with a little downward pressure.

POACHING

2 (6-ounce, 1-inch-thick) fish fillets

1. In a medium pot over medium heat, bring to a simmer enough water to cover fish by at least ½ inch.

2. Add herbs, spices, salt, citrus, aromatics like garlic and onion, or a few splashes of wine to the water while it's coming up to a simmer, if desired. It lends a subtle flavor but is not necessary.

3. Submerge fish, cover, and cook, 5 minutes.

4. Remove the pot from heat and keep covered undisturbed, 5 minutes or until an instant-read thermometer inserted into the thickest part of the fish reads 145°F. Fish will continue to cook.

5. Fish will be opaque and flake easily with a little downward pressure.

> **Nutrition for pan-seared fillet:** 260 calories, 440 mg omega-3s, 2 g saturated fat, 45 g protein, 0 g carbohydrates, 0 g fiber, 0 g added sugars, 650 mg potassium, 0.2 mg vitamin B6, 10 mcg folate, 3.2 mcg vitamin B12, 90 mg choline, 0 mcg lutein

> **Nutrition for poached fillet:** 220 calories, 410 mg omega-3s, 2 g saturated fat, 45 g protein, 0 g carbohydrates, 0 g fiber, 0 g added sugars, 650 mg potassium, 0.2 mg vitamin B6, 10 mcg folate, 3.2 mcg vitamin B12, 90 mg choline, 0 mcg lutein

TIPSY PRUNES & PORK

Wine-soaked prunes and pork is a traditional French bistro dish. The prunes shine in this simple yet luxurious dish. They offer powerful polyphenols, and the pork provides important B vitamins and a leaner cut is especially brain-healthy. A hearty serving of this dish is rich in protein, potassium, vitamin B6, vitamin B12, and choline and is a good source of fiber, vitamin E, and iron.

MIND foods: Whole grains, olive oil, wine

Yield: 2 (5-ounce pork with prunes and sauce) servings | **Time:** 50 minutes

12 ounces 1-inch-thick pork loin chop

½ teaspoon Diamond Crystal kosher salt

2 teaspoons ground coriander

1 teaspoon ground cumin

1 teaspoon smoked ground paprika

¼ teaspoon ground turmeric

¼ teaspoon freshly ground black pepper

1 tablespoon olive oil

½ teaspoon whole wheat flour

1 sprig flat leaf parsley, leaves only, chopped

ribbons of zest from a medium orange, to taste

TIPSY PRUNES & SAUCE

¼ cup port

¼ cup broth

⅓ cup packed prunes

¼ teaspoon ground cinnamon

¼ teaspoon Diamond Crystal kosher salt

1 tablespoon olive oil

½ teaspoons Dijon mustard

1. On a large rimmed plate, pat dry the pork loin chop. Season with ½ teaspoon of salt on all sides and rest 30 minutes on the counter.

2. In a small bowl, make the spice rub by stirring together the coriander, cumin, paprika, turmeric, and black pepper.

3. When the pork is done resting, heat 1 tablespoon of oil in a heavy-bottom pan, such as a cast-iron Dutch oven, on medium-high, 2 minutes. Meanwhile, pat the pork dry with paper towels, rub with flour on all sides, then follow with the spice rub.

4. Add the pork to the pan and sear, letting it cook undisturbed for 4 minutes. Next, holding the pork with kitchen tongs, sear the edges, holding 30 seconds per side, 2 minutes total. Return the pork to lie flat in the pot so that the seared side is now up. Cover and reduce the heat to medium-low and cook for an additional 5 to 6 minutes, or until an instant-read thermometer reads 145°F.

5. Move the tongs and the plate that held raw pork to the dishwasher or sink to avoid cross-contamination. Wash hands. Prep a clean plate with a foil tent. When the pork is done, transfer it to the plate and cover with the foil tent to rest 3 to 5 minutes.

6. For the sauce, bring the heat back up to medium-high. Add the port and scrape up any bits of fond on the bottom of the pot. Add the broth, prunes, cinnamon, and salt. Bring to a boil, then lower heat to a simmer to reduce sauce, about 5 minutes, stirring occasionally. Turn heat off and remove from heat. Set aside.

7. Move the pork to a cutting board, trim any visible fat, and slice the pork crosswise into even pieces about ¼ to ½ inch thick. Optional: slice at a slight diagonal, or bias cut, for presentation.

Transfer to a serving plate. Using a slotted spoon, transfer prunes to top of pork.

8. Whisk 1 tablespoon olive oil and Dijon into the pan until sauce thickens slightly; it will thicken more as it cools. Taste and adjust with more olive oil to soften flavors or more salt to bring flavors up. Spoon the sauce over the pork.

9. Garnish with parsley and strands of orange zest, to taste.

Notes: A citrus zester is different from a microplane, though they both get the zest off citrus well. A citrus zester will have small sharp holes (often 5) at one end that you drag across citrus peels to create long thin ribbons of zest that are perfect for garnishing.

Substitution options: Try replacing the tawny port with a dry red wine such as cabernet sauvignon, pinot noir, merlot, or tempranillo.

Level-up: Zest the orange directly over the pork just before eating to release its volatile oils onto the dish for a pleasant aroma.

> **Nutrition:** 520 calories, 150 mg omega-3s, 4 g saturated fat, 40 g protein, 37 g carbohydrates, 4 g fiber, 0 g added sugars, 1120 mg potassium, 1.4 mg vitamin B6, 0 mcg folate, 0.9 mcg vitamin B12, 110 mg choline, 300 mcg lutein

BASIC POACHED CHICKEN

Recipes don't get much simpler than this, but I'm including it here because I think it will be a workhorse of a recipe for you. You don't need to add lemon, or salt, or brine or do anything extra. Poaching is a gentle cooking method, yielding chicken that is tender and juicy. A serving provides half the day's protein and vitamin B6 and is a good source of choline.

MIND foods: Lean poultry
Yield: Makes 4 (3-ounce) servings | **Time:** 35–40 minutes

1 pound boneless skinless chicken
    breasts

1. Trim or pound chicken breasts to ¾ to 1 inch thickness and rest at room temperature 15 to 30 minutes.

2. In a medium pot with a tight-fitting lid, bring water to boil over high heat. There should be enough water to comfortably cover chicken breasts by at least a half inch when in a single layer.

3. When the water is boiling, add the chicken in a single layer and bring the water back to a boil, then cover, turn heat off immediately, and remove the pot from the heat source. Keep covered to hold steam in, 20 minutes. A little longer is OK, as this is a gentle cooking method.

4. When the chicken is done poaching and has an internal temperature of 165°F, transfer it to a cutting board and cut crosswise into ¾-inch slices, or transfer to a large mixing bowl and pull apart with 2 forks to create shreds.

Notes: The flavor is pure chicken. Enjoy it on its own or with your favorite sauce, add it to sandwiches, salads, and soups, or toss it with olive oil, a little sea salt, and your favorite spices.

Nutrition: 140 calories, 30 g omega-3s, 1 g saturated fat, 26 g protein, 0 g carbohydrates, 0 g fiber, 0 g added sugars, 380 mg potassium, 0.9 mg vitamin B6, 10 mcg folate, 0.2 mcg vitamin B12, 90 mg choline, 0 mcg lutein

KOREAN STIR-FRIED CHICKEN

A stir-fry is great way to use up odds and ends from the week's meals, from roasted veggies to whatever is about to be tossed from the produce drawers. This one is inspired by the Korean pantry ingredients of my youth. The spice level is mild, so everyone can enjoy. A serving is an excellent source of protein and vitamin B6, and a good source of vitamin D, potassium, and choline.

MIND foods: More vegetables, lean poultry, wine
Yield: 5 (¾-cup) servings | **Time:** 35–40 minutes

SAUCE

3 tablespoons soy sauce

1 tablespoon unseasoned rice wine

5 cloves garlic

1 inch ginger, unpeeled, with hard bits trimmed

1 tablespoon sesame oil

1 tablespoon gochujang

1 tablespoon light agave syrup

STIR-FRY

1 pound skinless boneless chicken breast, cut to 1-inch cubes

2 cups baby portobello mushrooms, quartered

1 medium carrot, peeled and cut into ⅛-inch matchsticks

½ large red or yellow bell pepper, cut into ⅛-inch matchsticks

1 tablespoon avocado oil

1½ cups broccoli florets

1 stalk green onion, sliced

1½ teaspoons toasted sesame seeds

1. Blend all the sauce ingredients in to a personal inverted blender, 3 seconds at a time, pausing to shake as needed, until garlic is minced, 10 to 15 seconds of blending total.

2. In a medium bowl, massage the chicken with 3 tablespoons of sauce. Set aside.

3. Heat a 10-inch wok over medium heat, 30 seconds. Add the avocado oil and heat for 30 to 90 seconds.

4. Add the chicken and cook for 2 minutes, flip, and cook for 2 minutes more.

5. Add the mushrooms and cook until they reduce, tossing occasionally, 5 minutes.

6. Add the carrots and cook, tossing occasionally, 1 minute.

7. Add the broccoli and remaining sauce and cook, tossing occasionally, 4 minutes.

8. Add the bell peppers and cook, tossing occasionally, 1 to 2 minutes, until just wilted. The broccoli will be cooked through at this point but not fully wilted.

9. Serve family style or divide between 4 plates. Enjoy with brown rice, a whole grain medley, or with roasted vegetables.

Notes: Korean stir-fry dishes often have loose pan drippings rather than a thick sauce. Rice does a good job of soaking it up.

A cast-iron wok will heat up quickly. Keep your eye on the pan, tossing as frequently as needed to avoid overcooking any of the ingredients. A high-walled sauté pan will also work.

Substitution options: Use any protein and vegetables you have on hand and mix and match. This is a very flexible recipe. The vegetables that need a little longer to cook should go in first.

Nutrition: 200 calories, 70 mg omega-3s, 1 g saturated fat, 23 g protein, 12 g carbohydrates, 2 g fiber, 0 g added sugars, 770 mg potassium, 0.9 mg vitamin B6, 30 mcg folate, 0.2 mcg vitamin B12, 90 mg choline, 60 mcg lutein

ALMOND & HERB-CRUSTED CHICKEN TENDERS

Almonds and Herbes de Provence elevate this take on chicken fingers. A serving is packed with protein, vitamin E, vitamin B6, vitamin B12, and choline and is a good source of fiber, potassium, and folate.

MIND foods: Nuts, whole grains, lean poultry

Yield: 3 (4-ounce chicken) servings | **Time:** 35–40 minutes

1 pound skinless boneless chicken breast (or precut tenders)
¼ teaspoon Diamond Crystal kosher salt
½ cup almonds
2 teaspoons Herbes de Provence
½ cup whole wheat panko bread crumbs

½ teaspoon gochugaru
½ teaspoon freshly ground black pepper
¼ teaspoon garlic powder
¼ cup Dijon mustard
1 green onion, sliced

1. Preheat the oven to 350°F for 15 minutes.

2. Pat the chicken dry and slice it into ¾-inch strips crosswise. Season with salt. Set aside.

3. In a mini food processor set to chop, pulse the almonds in 1-second intervals until they resemble coarse wet sand, about 1 minute.

4. In a large bowl, stir together the almonds, Herbes de Provence, panko bread crumbs, gochugaru, black pepper, and garlic powder.

5. To a medium bowl, add the Dijon mustard.

6. Pat the chicken dry again. Working one piece at a time, use your "wet hand" to coat a piece of chicken with Dijon mustard and transfer it to the bowl with dry ingredients. Use the your "dry hand" to press the dry mix onto the chicken, rotating as needed. Transfer to a rimmed sheet pan fitted with a wire rack. Repeat with remaining chicken.

7. Roast for 22 minutes, rest for 3 minutes. Garnish with green onion, if using. Enjoy with salad, in sandwiches, or with your favorite dipping sauce.

Substitution options: Instead of Herbes de Provence, you can sub Italian seasoning, or a mix of 2 or more of any of these: thyme, parsley, oregano, rosemary. To reduce spiciness, reduce the gochugaru or replace with paprika.

> **Nutrition:** 300 calories, 330 mg omega-3s, 2 g saturated fat, 39 g protein, 10 g carbohydrates, 3 g fiber, 0 g added sugars, 680 mg potassium, 3.8 mg vitamin B6, 70 mcg folate, 1 mcg vitamin B12, 400 mg choline, 120 mcg lutein

JUICY CHICKEN SHAWARMA PITA POCKETS

Chicken shawarma is enjoyed in the area of the Middle East near the eastern shores of the Mediterranean sea. The warm spices on the juicy chicken taste so good next to the refreshing yogurt sauce, cucumbers, and spring greens. Fill up a pita pocket for an excellent source of protein, vitamin E, iron, vitamin B6, vitamin B12, and choline. It's also a good source of fiber, potassium, and folate.

MIND foods: Leafy greens, more vegetables, whole grains, olive oil, lean poultry

Yield: 4 filled pita pockets | **Time:** 35–40 minutes

1 pound boneless skinless chicken breast, cut into 1-inch cubes

½ teaspoon salt

2 tablespoons Spice Blend

2 medium yellow onions, peeled, trimmed, and sliced into ¼-inch half moons

juice from 1 large lemon

½ cup olive oil

4 (7-inch) whole wheat pita halves, to serve

1 cup Cuke & Cumin Yogurt Dip (page 178), to serve

1 cup packed spring mix greens, to serve

1 (6-inch) Persian cucumber, sliced into ⅛-inch rounds, to serve

SPICE BLEND

1 tablespoon ground coriander

1 tablespoon ground cumin

1 tablespoon garlic powder

1 tablespoon gochugaru

1 tablespoon ground smoked paprika

1 tablespoon ground turmeric

1. Preheat the oven to 375°F.

2. In a large bowl, salt the chicken on all sides. Use kitchen tongs to mix. Keep the tongs in the bowl.

3. Add 2 tablespoons of the spice blend to coat the chicken on all sides, gently mixing with kitchen tongs.

4. Add the onions to the large bowl with the chicken, followed by lemon juice and olive oil. Use kitchen tongs to gently mix together.

5. Transfer the chicken-onion mixture onto a small quarter-sized sheet pan lined with a silicone baking mat.

6. Roast for 15 minutes. Check the internal temperature of the largest pieces with an instant-read thermometer. If it is below 165°F, rotate the pan and roast for an additional 5 minutes.

7. To each pita pocket, spread 2 to 3 tablespoons of yogurt dip on one side. Add ¼ cup packed spring mix and gently press to yogurt to keep it in place. Add about 3 chicken cubes and a few onions. Wedge in 7 to 10 cucumber slices on the other side of the chicken.

Notes: The generous amount of olive oil keeps the chicken juicy while roasting. Not all of it will be consumed and you will have about ¼ cup of liquid left on the baking pan. It can be saved to use the next day to cook eggs or vegetables.

You will have extra spice blend to use in other recipes such as Citrus Spiced Carrots (page 204).

Substitution options: Any small-seed cucumber will work in this recipe if Persian cucumbers are unavailable, including Korean, English, and Kirby cucumbers.

Level-up: While not necessary, the chicken-onion mix can be stored in the refrigerator for 3 hours or overnight to develop deeper flavors. Let it come to room temperature while the oven is preheating.

> **Nutrition:** 530 calories, 240 g omega-3s, 4 g saturated fat, 36 g protein, 40 g carbohydrates, 5 g fiber, 1 g added sugars, 890 mg potassium, 1.2 mg vitamin B6, 60 mcg folate, 0.5 mcg vitamin B12, 120 mg choline, 160 mcg lutein

WALNUT-CRUSTED SOY-SESAME CHICKEN

This flavorful walnut-crusted chicken recipe is elevated by east Asian flavors of soy, sesame, and ginger. Every bite is savory, tangy, and crunchy all at once. The coating ensures the chicken cooks to juicy perfection. Make this when you're craving flavor but running short on time. A serving is high in protein, vitamin D, vitamin B6 and choline and a good source of potassium and vitamin B12.

MIND foods: Nuts, whole grains, lean poultry

Yield: 3 (4-ounce chicken) servings | **Time:** 45 minutes

1 pound skinless boneless chicken breast (or precut tenders)
¼ teaspoon Diamond Crystal kosher salt
⅓ cup walnuts

3 tablespoons Dijon mustard
2 teaspoons low-sodium soy sauce
½ teaspoon toasted sesame oil
2 cloves garlic, roughly chopped

1 tablespoon minced fresh ginger
⅓ cup whole wheat panko bread crumbs

1 tablespoon gochugaru
1 green onion, sliced, to garnish (optional)

1. Preheat the oven to 350°F for 15 minutes.

2. Pat the chicken dry. Pound it to an even ¾-inch height. Season with salt on all sides. Set aside.

3. In a mini food processor set to chop, pulse the walnuts in 1-second intervals until they resemble coarse wet sand, about 1 minute. Transfer to a large bowl and wipe down the mini-food processor.

4. With the mini food processor set to puree, pulse the Dijon mustard, soy sauce, toasted sesame oil, garlic, and fresh ginger until smooth, scraping down sides as needed, 1 to 2 minutes. Transfer to a medium bowl.

5. To the large bowl with walnuts, add the panko bread crumbs and gochugaru. Stir to combine.

6. Pat the chicken dry again. Working one piece at a time, use your "wet hand" to coat a piece of chicken with the Dijon-soy mixture in the medium bowl, then transfer it to the large bowl with walnuts, bread crumbs, and gochugaru. Use your "dry hand" to press the dry mix onto the chicken, rotating as needed. Transfer to a rimmed sheet pan fitted with a wire rack. Repeat with remaining chicken.

7. Roast for 30 minutes, or until an instant-read thermometer reads 165°F. Rest for 3 minutes. Transfer to a cutting board and slice crosswise at a slight diagonal in ¾-inch increments. Transfer to a serving plate and garnish with green onion, if using. Enjoy with salad, pasta, or a whole grain salad.

Nutrition: 310 calories, 1070 mg omega-3s, 2 g saturated fat, 38 g protein, 15 g carbohydrates, 2.2 g fiber, 0 g added sugars, 770 mg potassium, 1.3 mg vitamin B6, 30 mcg folate, 0.3 mcg vitamin B12, 130 mg choline, 70 mcg lutein

Desserts

CHOCO-PEANUT BUTTER CUPS

These may remind you of a certain popular candy bar that rhymes with stickers. For a moment in the summer of 2023, a variation on these homemade copycats took over the internet. Mine are sized for built-in portion control but are plenty indulgent so that one is enough to satisfy your sweet tooth. You can feel good about the simple, wholesome ingredients.

MIND foods: Nuts

Yield: 24 (1 choco-peanut butter cup) servings | **Time:** 15 minutes, plus 1 hour to chill

¼ cup + 1 teaspoon peanut butter
1 (10-ounce) package bittersweet chocolate (60 percent cacao) baking wafers, divided

12 medjool dates, halved
½ cup chopped roasted and salted peanuts

1. Fit a silicone 24 mini-muffin pan into a 9 x 13-inch sheet pan. Set aside on a work surface.

2. In a microwave-safe dish, warm the peanut butter on high for 5 seconds. Stir. Repeat if needed until it's easy to drizzle. Set aside next to the sheet pan.

3. Next, melt and temper the chocolate. Fill a medium pot with about ¾ inch of water. Cover the pot with a large heat-safe glass mixing bowl so you can see when it starts to steam but it can't escape. Turn heat on low and keep water at a simmer or below. As soon as the steam touches the bowl, add a little more than half the baking chocolate and stir continuously. It's OK if it's a little difficult to stir, which is better than overheating the chocolate. When it's nearly all melted, with a handful of half-melted wafers still in the

mix, turn the heat off, take the bowl away from the heat, being careful no steam touches it, and add the rest of the baking chocolate. Stir vigorously until completely smooth. Transfer the bowl to your work surface.

4. Fill each mini muffin well with a scant teaspoon of melted chocolate.

5. Next, push half a medjool date, sticky side up, into each well so the chocolate comes up around the sides a little.

6. Next, add ½ teaspoon of peanut butter into each well, followed by ½ teaspoon of chopped peanuts.

7. Top with a scant teaspoon of melted chocolate and top evenly with the remaining chopped peanuts (~½ teaspoon per cup, but may be less). If you still have chocolate, you can drizzle some over the mini cups.

8. Transfer the tray into the freezer to flash freeze for at least an hour before popping the mini choco-peanut butter cups out. Store in an airtight container in the freezer for 1–3 months. Wait a few minutes after taking out of the freezer before eating.

Notes: Tempering chocolate seems complicated and there is some science involved, but as long as you keep the temperature low, you'll be fine. An instant-read thermometer or candy thermometer can help too. The goal is to get the chocolate to 89°F.

The silicone pan makes everything easier in this recipe. If unavailable, grease the wells of a metal mini muffin tin with oil before adding ingredients. Freeze for at least an hour before using a knife to loosen.

Nutrition: 130 calories, 0 mg omega-3s, 3 g saturated fat, 2 g protein, 16 g carbohydrates, 2 g fiber, 5 g added sugars, 120 mg potassium, 0.1 mg vitamin B6, 7 mcg folate, 0 mcg vitamin B12, 5 mg choline, 3 mcg lutein

ALMOND CITRUS CHOCOLATE BITES

Orange really loves chocolate, and they both love almonds, so these little dessert bites basically have it all. They are big on decadent indulgent flavor.

MIND foods: Nuts

Yield: 24 (1-bite) servings | **Time:** 1 hour 15 minutes, plus 1 hour to chill

24 Oven-Dried Citrus Circles (page 174)
1 (10-ounce) package bittersweet chocolate (60 percent cacao) baking wafers, divided
5¼ cups whole almonds

1. Make the Oven-Dried Citrus Circles. Use the 24 best ones for this dessert.

2. Meanwhile, clear a work area. Fit a silicone 24 mini-muffin pan onto a 9 x 13-inch sheet pan; set aside in your work area.

3. Next, melt and temper the chocolate. Fill a medium pot with about ¾ inch of water. Cover the pot with a large heat-safe glass mixing bowl so you can see when it starts to steam but it can't escape. Turn the heat to low and keep the water at a simmer or below. As soon as the steam touches the bowl, add a little more than half the baking chocolate and stir continuously. It's OK if it's a little difficult to stir, which is better than overheating the chocolate. When it's nearly all melted, with a handful of half-melted wafers still in the mix, turn the heat off, take the bowl away from the heat, being careful no steam touches it, and add the rest of the baking chocolate. Stir vigorously until completely smooth. Transfer the bowl to your work surface.

4. Fill each mini muffin well with a scant teaspoon of melted chocolate. Next, place 3 to 5 almonds in each well in a single layer. Top with another scant teaspoon of melted chocolate. Top with a citrus circle. Gently press the citrus circle into the chocolate so it adheres.

5. Transfer the tray into the freezer to flash freeze for at least an hour before popping the almond citrus chocolate bites out. Store in an airtight container in the freezer for 1 to 3 months. Wait a few minutes after taking out of the freezer before eating.

Notes: See notes about tempering in the Choco-Peanut Butter Cups recipe (page 230). One thing I'll add is that I've seen lots of recipes that use coconut oil. It's completely unnecessary if you melt the chocolate at a very low temperature so it doesn't overheat.

A semi-flexible mixing spatula works well for mixing the chocolate, but any mixing spoon will work.

Nutrition: 95 calories, 0 mg omega-3s, 3 g saturated fat, 2 g protein, 8 g carbohydrates, 2 g fiber, 5 g added sugars, 55 mg potassium, 0 mg vitamin B6, 4 mcg folate, 0 mcg vitamin B12, 4 mg choline, 15 mcg lutein

CREAMY NO-COOK PB&J MOUSSE

PB&J sounds basic, and this recipe is simple, but the taste and the look are elevated. Even better, there's no cooking involved, so this is perfect to make on a hot summer day or anytime you want a simple sweet treat.

MIND foods: Nuts

Yield: 2 (⅓-cup) servings | **Time:** 10 minutes

½ cup reduced fat plain Greek yogurt
2 tablespoons creamy peanut butter
½ teaspoon pure vanilla extract

2 tablespoons + 2 teaspoons Prune Puree (page 162), divided
pinch of Diamond Crystal kosher salt, divided
1 teaspoon cacao nibs, divided

1. In a medium bowl, mix together the yogurt, peanut butter, vanilla, and 2 tablespoons of Prune Puree until smooth.

2. To serve, divide "mousse" evenly into two dessert bowls such as ramekins, demi-coupe glasses, or small bowls. Add a teaspoon of Prune Puree in the center of each bowl and spiral from the center

out so it creates a swirl. Sprinkle a tiny pinch of salt over each bowl, then garnish with ½ teaspoon of cacao nibs each.

3. Enjoy right away or chill until ready to eat (it will get thicker when chilled).

Notes: Made ahead, the texture is even creamier after chilling.

Substitution options: If cacao nibs are unavailable, omit or use small dark chocolate chips or shavings.

> **Nutrition:** 185 calories, 20 mg omega-3s, 3 g saturated fat, 10 g protein, 15 g carbohydrates, 3 g fiber, 0 g added sugars, 310 mg potassium, 0.1 mg vitamin B6, 18 mcg folate, 0.2 mcg vitamin B12, 20 mg choline, 20 mcg lutein

SALGUSSAM (WALNUT-STUFFED APRICOTS)

This is a riff on a popular Korean treat that wraps walnuts in dried persimmon, but uses dried apricots, which are often easier to find in the United States.

MIND foods: Nuts

Yield: 4 (3-piece) servings | **Time:** 10 minutes, plus 1+ hours to freeze

9 dried apricots
12 walnut halves

1. Trim the top and bottom of the apricots. Save the trimmed ends. Set aside.

2. Using a paring knife, score an apricot lengthwise, being careful not to slice all the way through. Gently open up the apricot with the sticky side up, stretching it gently so it lies flat. Repeat with two more apricots. This can get sticky, so keep a towel nearby.

3. Slightly overlap the 3 apricot strips on a long side so they stick together. Further help them stick together by using four trimmed ends, sticky side down across the seams, perpendicular to the apricot strips. It should look like four "staples."

4. Flatten the apricot sheet further by placing a piece of parchment paper over the sticky surface and gently but firmly flatten it with a straight-walled glass, rolling pin, or the heel of your hand. This also helps the apricot pieces adhere to each other.

5. On a piece of plastic wrap that is at least 2 inches longer and wider than your apricot strip, lay the apricot sheet so a short side is facing you.

6. Next, lay a walnut half, flat side up, in the bottom left of the apricot sheet with a long edge facing you. Repeat on the bottom right of the apricot sheet.

7. Lay two more walnut halves, flat-side down, on top of the first set of walnut halves.

8. Carefully but as tightly as you can, roll the apricot sheet away from you to wrap the walnut in an apricot blanket until the apricot ends overlap. If needed, pinch the ends together so they stick.

9. Fold the plastic wrap, around the short ends and over the long end so it's sealed.

10. Gently but firmly compress the rolls to push the soft apricot flesh into the folds of the walnut without breaking the walnuts. Rolls will be about 2 inches long.

11. Repeat with the remaining apricots and walnuts, then place all the rolls in a freezer-safe container and freeze for at least an hour, ideally overnight.

12. When you're ready to enjoy, pull a roll out of the freezer and slice into 4 even ½-inch rounds. Enjoy with tea, as a snack, or as dessert. These also make nice homemade gifts.

Notes: In Korean, *salgu* means "apricots" and *ssam* means "wrap," which is where this treat gets its name.

Despite how long the instructions are, making these is quick work.

GREEK YOGURT WITH PORT WINE REDUCTION AND WALNUTS

This simple treat is inspired by a Greek dessert of yogurt, honey, and walnuts. This version adds a touch of vanilla to the thick and creamy yogurt base and tops it off with a decadent port wine reduction that gets its sweetness from the natural sugars from the wine. Plus, once you make the port wine reduction (which is super simple!), this comes together in under 5 minutes.

MIND foods: Nuts, wine

Yield: 1 (dessert) serving | **Time:** 40 minutes

¼ cup Greek yogurt (or other strained
    yogurt)
2 teaspoons port wine reduction
2 tablespoons chopped walnuts

PORT WINE REDUCTION INGREDIENTS

1½ cups tawny port wine
1½ teaspoons lemon zest, finely grated
    with a microplane
1½ teaspoons orange zest, finely
    grated with a microplane

1. In a medium pot, combine the port wine, lemon zest, and orange zest and bring up to a boil, then lower heat to a steady simmer. Simmer for 30 minutes or until the liquid is reduced to ¼ cup. The liquid should be thickened (it will thicken more as it cools too) and slowly drizzle off a spoon. Strain out the lemon and orange zest.

2. To an 8-ounce glass, such as a demi-coupe, add the yogurt, top with port wine reduction, then garnish with chopped walnuts.

Notes: This recipe calls for straining the lemon and orange zest from the port wine reduction, but don't toss it out. The zest is delicious in its own right and would make a lovely topping to any dessert. You can opt to leave it in for a more rustic reduction.

Substitution options: This would also be lovely with a few berries on top. And while the port wine reduction is a beautiful element of this dish, if you wanted a quicker version, you could replace it with pure maple syrup or honey.

Nutrition: 220 calories, 1150 mg omega-3s, 2 g saturated fat, 8 g protein, 12 g carbohydrates, 1 g fiber, 0 g added sugars, 200 mg potassium, 0.1 mg vitamin B6, 14 mcg folate, 0.2 mcg vitamin B12, 14 mg choline, 1 mcg lutein

Sips & Elixirs

TURMERIC WELLNESS SHOT

You may have seen pricey wellness shots in the grocery stores. They're simple to make at home. This turmeric wellness shot delivers bracing bold flavors, courtesy of anti-inflammatory curcumin, the antioxidant polyphenol in turmeric, and unfiltered apple cider vinegar. The black pepper increases the bioavailability of the curcumin by up to 2000 percent.

Yield: 1 wellness shot | **Time:** 2 minutes

¼ teaspoon ground turmeric
2 tablespoons tangerine juice, divided
1 teaspoon honey
1 teaspoon water

1 tablespoon unfiltered apple cider vinegar
tiny pinch of freshly ground black pepper
1 large ice cube

1. Into an 8-ounce wide-mouth glass, combine the turmeric and just enough tangerine juice to cover it. Whisk until smooth.

2. In a small microwave-safe bowl, combine the honey and water. Microwave for 5 to 7 seconds to dissolve honey.

3. Add the honey-water mixture, remaining tangerine juice, apple cider vinegar, and black pepper to the wide-mouth glass. Whisk to combine.

4. Add one large ice cube. Enjoy.

Notes: Bamboo whisks (chasen) can be found online for under $10. The recommended size and type of glass and ice cubes aren't essential to the recipe, though I think they'll provide a nice experience. Feel free to use the glassware and ice cubes you have available.

Substitution options: Try fresh lemon juice instead of apple cider vinegar. Try playing with less or more turmeric to adjust the bitterness to your palate. More turmeric will be more bitter.

Level-up: Chill your glass before adding ingredients. Place it in the freezer for 30 to 120 minutes. If short on time, fill the glass with ice and water for a few minutes, tossing (or using to water plants) before making this drink.

Nutrition: 40 calories, 0 mg omega-3s, 0 g saturated fat, 0 g protein, 10 g carbohydrates, 0 g fiber, 0 g added sugars, 90 mg potassium, 0 mg vitamin B6, 0 mcg folate, 0 mcg vitamin B12, 0 mg choline, 50 mcg lutein

ELDERBERRY SUNSET SPRITZ

Inspired by the pretty red and orange tequila sunrise cocktail, this zero-proof cocktail (aka mocktail) is for those times when you just want something fun and pretty to sip, without the hangover. The elderberry liquid adds a darker purply-red to this drink, so I'm calling it a "sunset" spritz instead of "sunrise."

MIND foods: Berries

Yield: 1 beverage | **Time:** 1 minute

2 ounces grapefruit sparkling water
2 ounces orange juice
1 teaspoon elderberry liquid

1. Into a champagne flute, pour the grapefruit sparkling water then the orange juice.

2. Tilt the glass slightly and spoon in the elderberry liquid down one side of the glass. Enjoy.

Notes: Elderberry liquid has no added sugar and is different from elderberry syrup. It can be found in health stores or online. If you can't find elderberry liquid, the syrup also works in this recipe because they are both heavier than the juice and sparkling water and will sink to the bottom to make the sunset ombré colors.

Substitution options: Try peach or mango juice instead of orange juice. Try plain sparkling water or other citrus or berry-flavored sparkling waters.

Level-up: Chill your champagne flute before adding ingredients. Place it in the freezer for 30 to 120 minutes. If you're short on time, fill the glass with ice and water for a few minutes, tossing (or using it to water plants) before making this drink.

> **Nutrition:** 45 calories, 0 mg omega-3s, 0 g saturated fat, 1 g protein, 11 g carbohydrates, 0 g fiber, 0 g added sugars, 110 mg potassium, 0 mg vitamin B6, 0 mcg folate, 0 mcg vitamin B12, 0 mg choline, 0 mcg lutein

WATERMELON-RASPBERRY COOLER

Did you know most watermelon in the United States is seedless and that it's available year-round? That means you can enjoy this watermelon mocktail anytime. The raspberry tempers and smooths out the crisp sweet watermelon to make this one cool quencher. This tall glass of freshness is also a surprisingly great source of fiber.

MIND foods: Berries
Yield: 1 mocktail | **Time:** 5 minutes

2 cups watermelon
½ cup frozen raspberries
1 tablespoon fresh lime juice

5 fresh mint leaves
¼ cup sparkling water

mini watermelon wedge, to garnish (optional)

lime wedge, to garnish (optional)

mint sprig, to garnish (optional)

fresh raspberry, to garnish (optional)

1. Place an 8 x 8-inch square of cheesecloth over a 5 to 6-inch fine-mesh strainer positioned over a large bowl.

2. Blend all ingredients except garnishes in a blender, then pour slowly over the cheesecloth. When most of the liquid has passed through, carefully gather up the cheesecloth by its corners and gently squeeze to extract additional liquid. Repeat if desired to remove more pulp.

3. Add ice to a 16-ounce glass, then pour mixture over ice. Top with up to ¼ cup sparkling water, to taste. Optional: pierce garnishes with a cocktail pick and place over the top of the glass.

Substitution options: For an alternate take on this sipper, skip the straining step and enjoy this as a smoothie.

Level-up: Large ice cubes melt more slowly and preserve the flavors of a mixed mocktail better. Smaller ice cubes will water it down more quickly, so if using smaller ice cubes, reduce or omit the sparkling water.

Nutrition: 100 calories, 90 mg omega-3s, 0 g saturated fat, 2 g protein, 25 g carbohydrates, 5 g fiber, 0 g added sugars, 350 mg potassium, 0.1 mg vitamin B6, 20 mcg folate, 0 mcg vitamin B12, 18 mg choline, 130 mcg lutein

PURPLE IS THE NEW PINK MOCKTAIL

The deep purple color of concord grape juice signals that there are antioxidant polyphenols inside, and it's a nonalcoholic way to enjoy many of the same antioxidants that are in wine.

Yield: 1 mocktail | **Time:** 5 minutes

¼ cup black tea, made with 2 tea bags and steeped for 10 minutes

¼ cup Concord grape juice

juice from 1 lemon

¼ cup pasteurized egg whites

1½ teaspoons light agave syrup (optional)

3 small red seedless grapes, for garnish (optional)

1. In a cocktail shaker or a large mason jar with a lid, add the black tea, concord grape juice, lemon juice, egg whites, and agave (if using) and seal, then shake for 10 seconds or until foam forms. If using a jar, use a large jar with room for the egg foam to expand.

2. Add 2 to 3 large ice cubes (or 5 to 10 regular ice cubes), re-seal and shake for another 5 to 10 seconds or until the shaker (or jar) is cold to the touch.

3. Strain into an 8-ounce demi-coupe or wine glass. Pierce grapes with a cocktail pick for a garnish, if using.

Notes: This mocktail uses a mixology technique of an initial dry shake (without ice) to help a nice egg foam form.

For a sipping drink that is pleasantly bitter, omit the agave and drink it straight up without ice, as written in the recipe. For a more refreshing sip, use the agave with the option to pour the mocktail into a glass over ice.

Substitution options: Try other darkly hued 100 percent juices, including tart cherry juice, cranberry juice, or blueberry juice. If sensitive to caffeine, try using a decaffeinated tea. For garnish, 3 blueberries also work well.

Level-up: Pre-chill your glass in the refrigerator, or by filling with ice while prepping your drink. Discard ice before pouring drink in.

Nutrition: 120 calories, 0 mg omega-3s, 0 g saturated fat, 7 g protein, 25 g carbohydrates, 1 g fiber, 0 g added sugars, 220 mg potassium, 0 mg vitamin B6, 12 mcg folate, 0.1 mcg vitamin B12, 0 mg choline, 20 mcg lutein

COCONUT WHISPER MOCKTAIL

This refreshing coconut-lime cooler has a nuanced whisper-of-coconut flavor combined with a fun foam and garnished with fresh mint for an inviting aroma. It's also a surprisingly good source of protein, thanks to the egg white foam.

Yield: 1 drink | **Time:** 5 minutes

¾ cup pure coconut water
juice from 1 lime
¼ cup pasteurized egg whites
1 fresh mint sprig, for garnish
   (optional)

1. In a cocktail shaker or a large mason jar with a lid, add the coconut water, lime juice, and egg whites, seal, then shake for 10 seconds or until foam forms. If using a jar, use a large jar with room for the egg foam to expand.

2. Add 2 to 3 large ice cubes (or 5 to 10 regular ice cubes), re-seal, and shake for another 5 to 10 seconds or until the shaker (or jar) is cold to the touch.

3. Strain into a 10- to 12-ounce glass filled with ice. Garnish with a fresh mint sprig, if using.

> **Nutrition:** 70 calories, 0 mg omega-3s, 0 g saturated fat, 8 g protein, 9 g carbohydrates, 2 g fiber, 0 g added sugars, 410 mg potassium, 0.1 mg vitamin B6, 10 mcg folate, 0.1 mcg vitamin B12, 3 mg choline, 0 mcg lutein

BORICHA (ROASTED BARLEY TEA)

This caffeine-free tea is enjoyed in Korea and neighboring countries. It has a mild nutty and toasty flavor that is comforting on a cold day. Better yet, antioxidants and some of the minerals in barley make their way into the tea. If you eat the roasted and soaked barley when you're done with the tea, you'll also enjoy a good source of fiber.

MIND foods: Whole grains
Yield: 4 (¾-cup) servings | **Time:** 30 minutes, plus 30 minutes to cool

½ cup dry barley
4 cups water

1. Add dry barley to a 10-inch cast-iron pan in a single layer over medium-low heat, swirling occasionally for 10 to 15 minutes until toasted but not burnt. Cool completely (30+ minutes) and store in an airtight container in a cool, dry place until ready to use.

2. Bring 4 cups of water to a boil, add the barley, stir, then reduce heat to a simmer and simmer for 10 minutes. Tea will be a light golden-honey color.

3. Enjoy hot or chilled.

Notes: For a quicker tea, once roasted barley is cool, use a spice grinder to break it into smaller pieces until it resembles coarse sand. Anytime you want to enjoy this tea, add a teaspoon or more to a mug and fill with 6 to 8 ounces of hot water and steep for 3 to 5 minutes. No need to strain the barley. It can even be eaten, if desired.

Because this tea is a simple infusion with 2 ingredients, the quality of those ingredients matters. Use the best-quality barley and cleanest water you have available to you.

> **Nutrition:** 80 calories, 30 mg omega-3s, 0 g saturated fat, 3 g protein, 17 g carbohydrates, 4 g fiber, 0 g added sugars, 100 mg potassium, 0.1 mg vitamin B6, 0 mcg folate, 0 mcg vitamin B12, 10 mg choline, 40 mcg lutein

PART THREE

Tips and Tools

The tips and tools in this chapter are meant to support you as you take action toward brain health and Alzheimer's prevention. It includes the top expert-backed lifestyle recommendations from the National Institute on Aging and the Global Council on Brain Health, including the six pillars of brain health and the crucial role of lifestyle factors in maintaining cognitive reserve in late life.

Practical resources like tip sheets and starter guides provide actionable advice on preparing your kitchen for the MIND diet, utilizing MIND foods in creative ways, and identifying top sources of plant proteins, omega-3s, fiber-rich beans, sustainable seafood, and brain-healthy foods outside the MIND diet.

You'll also be equipped with ideas for simple snack pairings, seasonal food recommendations, hydration tips, an at-a-glance MIND diet overview, and trackers for monitoring whole grains and foods to limit. Finally, we address cultural adaptations of the MIND diet and a robust section on frequently asked questions.

CHAPTER 9
LIFESTYLE RECOMMENDATIONS FOR BRAIN HEALTH

A healthy diet and lifestyle have so many benefits. This chapter reviews recommendations from Alzheimer's disease experts in collaboration with the National Institute on Aging, and the Global Council on Brain Health.

Together these lifestyle strategies may help people build cognitive reserve, which powers the brain's ability to adapt and may explain why some people's brains are better at resisting decline. A brain with a strong cognitive reserve has the resources to help defend itself against aging and disease, like a retirement account that can handle any unexpected expenses that come up. A strong brain reserve will help people preserve their ability to focus, multitask, hold onto information, find words, and navigate the small and large challenges of their daily lives.

National Institute on Aging Dietary & Lifestyle Guidelines for the Prevention of Alzheimer's Disease

The following seven diet and lifestyle guidelines to prevent Alzheimer's disease are the result of an expert roundtable meeting hosted by the National Institute on Aging. Notably, the roundtable included lead MIND diet researcher Dr. Morris. The scientists dutifully note that the scientific evidence is not yet complete, and that they compiled these practical everyday guidelines using the precautionary principle (i.e., better safe than sorry), using the best evidence available to them.

Many of the recommendations should look familiar, as they're in line with diet and lifestyle advice for the general public, such as to eat more vegetables and exercise regularly. Other recommendations are more specific to the research on cognitive decline and Alzheimer's disease, such as avoiding aluminum.

Guidelines At-a-Glance

1. Avoid saturated and trans fat.
2. Most of what you eat should be vegetables, legumes, fruits, and whole grains.
3. Eat food, and not supplements, for vitamin E.
4. Find a good source of vitamin B12 every day.
5. If you take a multivitamin, don't go overboard on iron and copper.
6. Avoid aluminum, which can be in cookware, antacids, baking powder, and other products.
7. Walk briskly for 40 minutes every other day.

This book has covered guidelines one through four, and guideline seven is self-explanatory, so the below will briefly discuss guidelines five and six.

Guideline 5: Avoid Excessive Iron and Copper in Supplements

Iron and copper are essential trace minerals important for normal brain function and good health. However, some studies suggest that excessive intake of these minerals, especially in combination with a diet high in saturated fat, contributes to cognitive problems and increased risk of Alzheimer's disease. As is common in nutrition, getting the right amount of any nutrient matters. Too little or too much can put you out of balance and have negative effects. Too much iron and copper can produce oxidative stress in the brain. Supplements are meant to fill nutritional gaps not met by food, so before taking a supplement with high levels of iron or copper, it would be helpful to know your status.

In the United States, infants, teen girls, pregnant women, and perimenopausal women are at risk of not getting enough iron, as are frequent blood donors, people with cancer, people with heart failure, and people with gastrointestinal disorders or past gastrointestinal surgery that disrupts absorption. But some people may be getting too much. One study in 1,106 older white adults found they are more likely to get more iron than needed. Some people have a genetic predisposition to absorb iron (called hereditary hemochromatosis) that puts them at risk for iron overload. The recommended amount of daily intake of iron for adults 51 years and older is 8 milligrams.

Copper deficiency is rare in the US, but more common in people with celiac disease because it disrupts nutrient absorption, and people who take a lot of zinc because it interferes with absorption too. Finally, people with a rare disease called Menkes disease are also at risk of poor copper absorption. Most Americans get all the copper they need from food.

Bottomline: Unless specifically guided by a health professional familiar with your individual needs, it's best to choose foods first over supplements to meet iron and copper recommendations. For supplements, look for those that have minimal to no iron and copper, or at least less than 100 percent of the Daily Value.

Guideline 6: Avoid Aluminum

The role of aluminum in Alzheimer's disease is controversial. Some researchers call for caution, while many experts agree that there is not enough evidence to say it clearly increases the risk for Alzheimer's disease. Aluminum, at high enough levels, has known neurotoxic potential. Aluminum has been found in the brains of people with Alzheimer's disease, and studies in Europe have observed higher rates of Alzheimer's disease in areas where the tap water was higher in aluminum.

Aluminum has no role in human biology, so there is no downside to avoiding exposure. In an abundance of caution, exposure can be minimized until the science has progressed. Aluminum is in some brands of baking powder, antacids, hemorrhoid medication, and other over-the-counter medicines; boxed cake mixes; deodorants and antiperspirants; douches; processed cheese; pickles; toothpaste; and table salts. As a food additive, aluminum is used as a firming agent in pickled products, as a pH-adjusting part of baking powder in bakery products, as emulsifying agents in processed cheese spread, and in food colorings.

Bottom line: In an abundance of caution, aluminum can be avoided in common household items by looking for it in the ingredients list of packaged items.

The National Institute on Aging (NIA) has more general lifestyle guidelines to improve overall health and well-being to lower the risk of conditions that may increase the risk of Alzheimer's disease, such as heart disease and diabetes.

- Healthy diet
- Physical activity
- Healthy weight
- No smoking

The NIA also recommends that older adults participate in activities for social engagement and mental stimulation. Some examples are below.

Social Activities

- Attend the theater or a sporting event.
- Travel with a group of friends.
- Visit family and friends.
- Serve meals at a soup kitchen.
- Volunteer at a local animal shelter, school, library, or hospital.

Mental Stimulation

- Take a cooking, art, or computer class.
- Form or join a book club.
- Learn how to play a musical instrument.
- Play cards or other games with friends.
- Sing in a community choral group.

6 Pillars of Brain Health from the Global Council on Brain Health

The Global Council on Brain Health (GCBH) has outlined six pillars of brain-healthy behaviors.[38] The GCBH is an independent consortium of scientists, health professionals, and policy experts

---

38   AARP, "Staying Sharp's Six Pillars of Brain Health," last accessed June 18, 2024, https://stayingsharp.aarp.org/about/brain-health/the-science.

worldwide who are working to improve people's ability to think and reason as they age, including memory, perception, and judgement.

1. **Eat well**—Eat a healthy, balanced diet. What we eat has direct and indirect effects on cognitive function and our mental and emotional well-being. Aging makes it more difficult to meet nutrient needs due to several factors—physical, metabolic, as well as psychosocial—that can impact quality of life. For all these reasons, accessible, nutrient-rich foods are especially important. The MIND diet is one approach, and is specifically designed to support brain health.

2. **Move more**—Find ways to move throughout the day. Aim for two and a half hours per week. Go for variety, including strength, endurance, balance, and flexibility exercises. This preserves the structural integrity of neurons and brain volume. It also helps maintain functional strength needed for independent living.

3. **Sleep soundly**—Stick to a regular sleep ritual that gives you seven to eight hours of good quality sleep every night. Sleep is when the brain does routine metabolic waste clean-up. Try to wake up and go to sleep around the same time each day, whether weekday, weekend, or on vacation.

4. **Make space to process life's stresses**—A stable schedule can help. Find activities that support your mental health. For many people, this is a joyful movement practice or time outdoors. Large-scale studies have found that a healthy diet supports better mental health outcomes. Consult a mental health professional for cases of ongoing or severe stress and anxiety.

5. **Socialize**—Keep in touch with friends and family. Super agers report more social connections, and past research has linked psychological wellbeing with a lower risk of

Alzheimer's. Being tied to something larger than yourself is also associated with better mental health.

6. **Keep your brain active**—Activate your mind. Never stop learning. Explore new interests and hobbies. It keeps the brain plastic and adaptable.

Lifestyle Factors for Cognitive Reserve in Late Life

Results from a 2024 study not only support these recommendations, they find that higher healthy lifestyle scores protected memory and cognition in older adults, even when their brains had common signs in the brain related to dementia, such as beta-amyloid plaques, tau tangles, Lewy body, and vascular disease. This is according to a study published in the *Journal of the American Medical Association for Neurology*, with autopsy data from 754 older adults (average age at death was 90 years) who were followed for more than 20 years.[39] The protective factors were a MIND diet score above 7.5, not smoking, at least 150 minutes of physical activity each week, limited alcohol intake, and stimulating brain activities such as reading, visiting museums, or playing games like cards, checkers, crosswords, or puzzles.

Bottom line: Eat well, move more, sleep soundly, manage stress, socialize, engage the brain, and don't smoke.

---

39 Dhana 2024.

CHAPTER 10
TIP SHEETS

Starter Tips to Get Your Kitchen MIND Diet Ready

Though the MIND diet is fairly straightforward and often celebrated for its simplicity, starting something new always has its challenges. Here are my top tips for getting your kitchen ready to make MIND diet meals and snacks. I hope these tips set you up for success, take some of the guesswork out of getting started, or at the very least, save you some time.

1. Look for prewashed salad greens so you don't have to think twice about adding a handful of leafy greens to your next meal, snack, soup, salad, or smoothie.

2. Keep the freezer stocked with leafy green vegetables, other vegetables, and berries.

3. Keep frozen seafood in stock. It cooks almost as quickly as fresh or thawed. I offer two methods in the recipes section.

4. Include some tinned seafood in your meals. They can be so delicious, they have a long shelf life, and they're very convenient. Try my smoked trout recipes (page 166), which use tinned smoked trout. Seafood also comes in jars, pouches, and tubes.

5. Store your nuts in the refrigerator or freezer to make them last longer. Stock up on a variety, starting with walnuts, almonds, peanuts, and their nut butters.

6. Stock the pantry with canned beans. Simply rinse before using to remove residue and as much sodium as possible. Look for low-sodium options and BPA-free packaging.

7. Look for whole grains marketed as "10-minute" versions to cut down on prep time, including 10-minute barley, farro, or bulgur.

8. Try fonio or whole wheat couscous, which are naturally quick-cooking whole grains that are done after five minutes of steaming in a covered pot.

9. Keep regular oats in stock. They cook quickly and can even be eaten raw, making them a good choice for quick breakfasts, overnight oats, and No-Bake Granola Balls (recipe on page 170).

10. Batch cook whole grains and freeze some for a later day. Frozen grains reheat nicely. They often just need a splash of water, then can be reheated, covered, in a microwave.

11. Don't be afraid to cook with extra-virgin olive oil (EVOO). Newer research suggests smoke point isn't the best indicator of an oil's performance, and has shown that EVOO has strong oxidative stability that can hold up sautéing, pan frying, roasting, and baking despite having a moderate smoke point.[40] The recipes in this book keep temperatures below 400°F, so you'll rarely if ever reach olive oil's smoke point of 350°–410°F regardless. The times you'll want to choose other oils are for flavor or cost.

---

40   De Alzaa et al., "Evaluation of Chemical and Physical Changes in Different Commercial Oils during Heating," *Acta Scientific Nutritional Health* 2, no .6 (2018): 2–11.

12. Choose boneless skinless chicken breasts and turkey cutlets, as they are the leanest poultry choices. For ground poultry, look for 90 to 95 percent lean.

13. Grocery store rotisserie chicken is convenient and very versatile. Remove the skin and visible fat before adding to recipes.

14. If you enjoy pork, choose pork tenderloin or boneless pork sirloin roast, both of which are American Heart Association Heart-Check Mark Certified foods.

15. The wine recommendation is optional. If drinking, it should be kept to one glass a day (5 ounces).

16. Ways to include wine in your diet without the alcohol are using wine-based vinegars in dressings, cooking with wine (e.g., sauces, poaching liquid, and reductions), or drinking nonalcoholic wine.

Top 10 Untraditional Ways to Use MIND foods

The MIND diet celebrates wholesome, natural, simple foods. That doesn't mean it has to be boring. On the contrary, here are 10 new ways to think about the classic foods in the MIND diet.

1. Black bean brownies are fudgy, delicious, and flourless. Pureed black beans replace flour and offer more phytonutrients and fiber. Stealth-health at its best. No one will ever guess the secret ingredient is black beans.

2. Leafy greens aren't just for salads; try them in smoothies. Blend them with your favorite frozen fruit, and you may not even notice there's a vegetable in your glass; or, load up on the leafy greens portion and combine with ginger and apples for a veggie-forward green juice.

3. Add silken soft tofu to smoothies and soups to make them rich and creamy without the cream. The mild flavor of tofu incorporates seamlessly into sweet and savory dishes alike. It'll also boost the plant protein in any meal.

4. Fish for breakfast may sound unusual to some, but give it a try. Mash tinned smoked trout in extra-virgin olive oil and combine with diced tomatoes. Top toast.

5. Eat eggs for lunch or dinner. We're used to eggs equaling breakfast, but it's a rule that's meant to be broken. Enjoy a veggie scramble, omelet, frittata, or egg sandwich for lunch or dinner as a quick and convenient way to add a serving of vegetables and/or whole grains to your day.

6. Make cauliflower into rice or couscous by cutting a head of cauliflower into quarters, removing the hard core and stem, and chopping until the pieces are your preferred size of rice or couscous (or give it a rough chop and add the pieces into a food processor to pulse briefly until the consistency you prefer is achieved). Heat for five to seven minutes with extra-virgin olive oil over medium heat for a healthy side dish.

7. Grilled berries make for a decadent dessert with no added sugar. Simply choose your favorite berries and wrap them in a parchment-paper-lined sheet of foil, or try adding lemon zest and balsamic vinegar to your berry mix for more complex flavors. Grill for about five minutes.

8. Breakfast rice porridge, fonio, or oatmeal works surprisingly well as a savory dish. Try steel cut oats topped with kimchi, a poached egg, and green onions; or, enjoy with shredded chicken and your favorite salsa.

9. Use veggies instead of pasta (or start by replacing half the pasta)—not because there's anything wrong with pasta—just

as a fun way to add more vegetables into meals. Spaghetti squash can step in for long spaghetti noodles, and long, flat slices of zucchini can stand in for lasagna pasta.

10. Add nut butters to smoothies, oatmeal, and yogurt for a rich, creamy flavor and to add some protein and healthy fat too.

Top 10 Plant Proteins

Many plant protein foods are affordable, sustainable, and delicious. Here are 10 great options to try, each with at least 5 grams of protein per serving.

1. Firm tofu—11 g per half cup
2. Hemp seeds—10 g per ounce (3 tablespoons)
3. Kamut wheat—10 g per cup (cooked)
4. Edamame – 9 g per half cup (cooked)
5. White beans—9 g per half cup (cooked)
6. Quinoa—8 g per cup (cooked)
7. Black beans—8 g per half cup (cooked)
8. Peanuts—7 g per ounce (¼ cup)
9. Wild rice—7 g per cup (cooked)
10. Buckwheat groats—6 g per cup (cooked)

Top Five Surprising Sources of Protein

Most foods have some protein in them, and they all contribute to your overall daily intake. The following foods contain a high percentage of protein, though serving sizes don't always mean it adds up to a huge amount. Both percent protein and grams of protein per serving are provided so you can make educated choices.

- Spirulina, dried—57 percent protein (4 g/tablespoon)
- Peanut flour, low-fat—34 percent protein (4 g/2 tablespoons)
- Gim (dried laver seaweed)—31 percent protein (1.5 g/10 sheets)
- Pumpkin seeds—30 percent protein (8 g/¼ cup)
- Wheat germ—27 percent protein (5 g/3 tablespoons)

Top Whole Plant Food Sources of Omega-3s

Plant-based omega-3s (ALAs) are essential and must come from food because the body cannot create them on its own. ALA can be converted to the types of omega-3s in seafood (EPA, then DHA). The Institute of Medicine recommends that women get at least 1.1 grams of plant-based omega-3s a day and that men get at least 1.6 grams per day. Needs are higher for pregnant and breastfeeding women, and lower for younger children.

1. Perilla seeds 3.8 g/tablespoon
2. Walnuts 2.6 g/ounce
3. Chia seeds 1.8 g/tablespoon
4. Flaxseed 1.6 g/tablespoon
5. Mature soybeans, roasted, 1.5 g/Half cup

6. Hemp seeds, 1g/tablespoon

7. Edamame, prepared, 0.3 g/Half cup

Top Seafood Sources of Omega-3s

The *Dietary Guidelines for Americans 2020–2025* notes that an average of 250 milligrams/day omega-3s from seafood improves heart health for people with or without heart disease. The American Heart Association recommends 1 gram a day for people with coronary heart disease. Choose a variety of seafood for omega-3s and lean protein. Below are options organized by omega-3 level per 3-ounce serving.

1000+ mg

- Arctic char
- Anchovies
- Herring
- Mackerel (Atlantic and Pacific)
- Oysters (Pacific)
- Black cod (Sablefish)
- Salmon (Atlantic and Chinook)
- Sardines
- Whitefish

500–1000 mg

- Barramundi
- Mussels
- Salmon (chum, coho, pink, and sockeye)
- Sea bass
- Squid (calamari)
- Trout
- Tuna (albacore)

250–500 mg

- Alaskan pollock
- Crab
- Flounder/sole
- King mackerel
- Rockfish
- Snapper
- Sturgeon
- Tuna (skipjack, canned)

<250 mg

- Catfish
- Clams
- Cod
- Crayfish
- Grouper
- Haddock
- Halibut
- Lobster
- Mahi mahi
- Scallops
- Shrimp
- Tilapia
- Tuna (yellowfin)

Top 21 Best Sustainable Seafood Choices

Sustainable seafood is well-managed and caught or farmed in ways with minimal environmental harm to habitats or other wildlife. The options below have been vetted by the Monterey Bay Aquarium and are current as of 2024. For the most up-to-date information, visit seafoodwatch.org. Sources with 500+ mg EPA+DHA omega-3s are in bold.

1. Abalone (farmed)
2. **Anchovy** (Spain, Bay of Biscay)
3. **Arctic char**
4. **Bass** (farmed, US)
5. Catfish (farmed, US)
6. Clams (farmed)
7. Pacific cod (Alaska)
8. King crab (Alaska)
9. Lionfish (US)
10. **Mussels** (farmed)
11. Oysters (farmed)

12. Rockfish (US)

13. **Salmon, chinook/king** (farmed, New Zealand)

14. Sanddab (US)

15. Scallops (farmed)

16. Shrimp (farmed, US)

17. **Squid** (California)

18. Sturgeon (farmed, US)

19. **Trout** (farmed, US)

20. Tuna, albacore/white (troll or pole and line)

21. Tuna, skipjack/chunk light (Pacific troll or pole and line)

Choosing Fish Lower in Mercury

Fish provides brain-healthy omega-3s, vitamin B12, vitamin D, selenium, iron, zinc, iodine, and choline, as well as a source of lean protein. There are many options to choose from while minimizing exposure to mercury. This list is from FDA.gov/fishadvice.

Best Choices: Go for one to three servings per week

- Anchovy
- Atlantic croaker
- Atlantic mackerel
- Black sea bass
- Butterfish
- Catfish
- Clam
- Cod
- Crab
- Crawfish
- Flounder
- Haddock
- Hake
- Herring
- Lobster, American and spiny
- Mullet
- Oyster
- Pacific chub mackerel
- Perch, freshwater and ocean
- Pickerel
- Plaice
- Pollock
- Salmon
- Sardine
- Scallop

- Shad
- Shrimp
- Skate
- Smelt
- Sole
- Squid

- Tilapia
- Trout, freshwater
- Tuna, canned light (includes skipjack)
- Whitefish
- Whiting

Good Choices: Go for one serving per week

- Bluefish
- Buffalofish
- Carp
- Chilean sea bass/ Patagonian toothfish
- Grouper
- Halibut
- Mahi mahi/dolphinfish
- Monkfish
- Rockfish
- Sablefish

- Sheepshead
- Snapper
- Spanish mackerel
- Striped bass (ocean)
- Tilefish (Atlantic Ocean)
- Tuna, albacore/white tuna, canned and fresh/frozen
- Tuna, yellowfin
- Weakfish/seatrout
- White croaker
- Pacific croaker

Choices to Limit: Highest mercury levels, avoid or eat sparingly

- King mackerel
- Marlin
- Orange roughy
- Shark

- Swordfish
- Tilefish (Gulf of Mexico)
- Tuna, bigeye

Top 10 Fiber-Rich Beans

Meeting daily fiber goals are much easier with beans on the menu. All beans are healthy choices and offer good nutrition. The beans on this list are excellent sources of fiber, providing at least 5 grams of fiber per Half cup cooked serving, or 20 percent of the Daily Value (25 grams) for fiber.

1. Navy beans—10 g fiber, 130 calories
2. Small white beans—9 g fiber, 130 calories
3. Cranberry (Roman) beans—9 g fiber, 130 calories
4. Chickpeas (garbanzo beans)—8 g fiber, 180 calories
5. Pinto beans—8 g fiber, 120 calories
6. Lima beans—7 g fiber, 110 calories
7. Great northern beans—6 g fiber, 150 calories
8. White beans—6 g fiber, 150 calories
9. Kidney beans—6 g fiber, 110 calories
10. Mature Soybeans—5 g fiber, 150 calories

Top Non-MIND Diet Brain-Healthy Foods

These foods aren't part of the core MIND diet but offer many valuable nutrients that are in line with a brain-healthy eating pattern. The below foods contain many brain-healthy nutrients and bioactives, and can be enjoyed in addition to the core MIND diet foods, even if they don't fall neatly into one of its categories.

1. Avocado
2. Cacao
3. Chia seeds

4. Coffee

5. Eggs

6. Flaxseed, ground

7. Green tea

8. Hemp seeds

9. Fermented foods

10. Perilla seeds

11. Prunes

12. Spices, especially turmeric, chilis

Top 10 Simple Snack Pairings

Eating doesn't have to be complicated. In fact, sometimes there's nothing nicer or more nutritious than the simplest of dishes. Here are 10 ideas for MIND-friendly snacks that are easy, healthy, and so delicious.

1. Fresh apricot with 14 walnut halves
   MIND foods: Nuts
   Nutrition: 180 calories, 13 g total fat, 2 g saturated fat, 6 g protein, 12 g carbohydrates, 4 g fiber

2. Half cup of halved strawberries with 23 almonds
   MIND foods: Berries, nuts
   Nutrition: 200 calories, 16 g total fat, 1 g saturated fat, 7 g protein, 11 g carbohydrates, 4 g fiber

3. A slice of 100 percent whole wheat toast topped with a quarter of a small avocado, a squeeze of fresh lemon juice, sprinkled with chili pepper flakes and good quality salt
   MIND foods: Whole grains
   Nutrition: 120 calories, 6 g total fat, 1 g saturated fat, 4 g protein, 14 g carbohydrates, 4 g fiber

4. 15 baby carrots drizzled with 2 teaspoons extra-virgin olive oil and 1 teaspoon balsamic vinegar, sprinkled with pepper
   MIND foods: Vegetables, olive oil
   Nutrition: 150 calories, 9 g total fat, 1 g saturated fat, 1 g protein, 15 g carbohydrates, 4 g fiber

5. Chopped ripe medium tomato topped with a quarter cup of tuna fish, drizzled with 2 teaspoons of extra-virgin olive oil, finished with fresh lemon juice and pepper
   MIND foods: Fish, olive oil
   Nutrition: 150 calories, 10 g total fat, 1 g saturated fat, 11 g protein, 5 g carbohydrates, 1 g fiber

6. 3 cups air-popped popcorn, drizzled with extra-virgin olive oil and dusted with dried herbs
   MIND foods: Whole grains, olive oil
   Nutrition: 170 calories, 10 g total fat, 1 g saturated fat, 3 g protein, 19 g carbohydrates, 3 g fiber

7. Half cup of cucumber slices combined with a tablespoon of champagne vinegar and pepper
   MIND foods: Vegetables
   Nutrition: 10 calories, 0 g total fat, 0 g saturated fat, 0 g protein, 1 g carbohydrates, 0 g fiber

8. A cup of baby arugula with five sliced strawberries and a tablespoon of balsamic vinaigrette
   MIND foods: Leafy greens, berries, olive oil
   Nutrition: 70 calories, 4 g total fat, 1 g saturated fat, 1 g protein, 7 g carbohydrates, 2 g fiber

9. Half cup of blueberries mixed with a quarter cup of granola, drizzled with a teaspoon of extra-virgin olive oil
   MIND foods: Berries, whole grains, olive oil
   Nutrition: 190 calories, 6 g total fat, 1 g saturated fat, 3 g protein, 33 g carbohydrates, 3 g fiber

10. Crudités, including 3-inch sticks of carrots (4), red bell pepper (8), and celery (4), with a tablespoon of Dijon mustard

MIND foods: Vegetables

Nutrition: 50 calories, 1 g total fat, 0 g saturated fat, 2 g protein, 9 g carbohydrates, 3 g fiber

What's in Season

Foods at peak season in your local area are at an ideal stage of quality, taste, and price. This holds true from produce to seafood. For the United States, here's a quick abbreviated guide to what kinds of MIND foods are at their best in each season. It's not comprehensive: the best way to understand what's in season in your specific region is to visit a local farmer's market (https://ams.usda.gov/local-food-directories/farmersmarkets).

Frozen and Canned

Frozen and canned goods are good ways to enjoy foods that have been preserved at peak season. Just make sure they're in a BPA-free container.

Winter

- Root vegetables and hardy cooking greens like collards and kale
- Mushrooms, onions and leeks, potatoes, sweet potatoes and yams, turnips, winter squash
- Northern hemisphere olive oils

Spring

- Strawberries and more delicate greens, from lettuce to string beans and asparagus
- Broccoli, cabbage, green beans, lettuce, mushrooms, onions and leeks, peas, spinach
- Northern hemisphere olive oils

Summer

- Berries in general and delicate salad greens
- Blackberries, blueberries, cherries, raspberries, strawberries
- Wild salmon
- Beets, bell peppers, corn, cucumbers, eggplant, garlic, green beans, lima beans, mushrooms, peas, radishes, summer squash, and zucchini
- Southern hemisphere olive oils

Fall

- Hardy vegetables like broccoli and brussels sprouts
- Beets, broccoli, brussels sprouts, carrots, cauliflower, garlic, ginger, mushrooms, parsnips, pumpkins, sweet potatoes and yams, winter squash
- Cranberries
- Southern hemisphere olive oils

Always in Season

- Dried whole grains
- Nuts
- Dried beans
- Wine
- Olive oil
- Poultry

14 Ways to Hydrate

To prevent dehydration, the National Academies of Medicine recommends that older women consume about 11.4 cups of total water per day, and men consume 15.6 cups of total water per day. We know from diet studies that about 20 percent of our total water should be coming from food, which means women should aim to drink about 9 cups of water a day and men should aim to drink about 13 cups of water per day. Individual needs may vary based on health conditions, physical activity levels, excessive heat, or sweating.

Even though the recommendations are for "water," that doesn't necessarily mean plain water. It can be water in that is in berries, leafy greens, cucumbers, melons, and soups. Coffee and tea count toward fluid intake, even though they were once thought of as diuretics (that has been debunked, and these drinks are OK when consumed at moderate levels of no more than 4 cups per day). The water intake is greater than any diuretic effect.

With all that in mind, here are 14 ways to hydrate through foods and drinks:

1. Plain water
2. Smoothies
3. Tea
4. Berries
5. Cucumbers
6. Sparkling water with citrus zest, fresh ginger, cucumber, or crushed mint
7. Watermelon
8. Milk
9. Fruit or vegetable juice
10. Coffee

11. Soup or broth

12. Frozen or fresh grapes

13. Set calendar reminders to hydrate

14. Anchor fluid intake to another habit; for example, drink a glass of water as soon as you wake up

A 2023 study found that poor hydration may speed up biological aging and increase the risk of chronic disease and premature death. This was an observational study that followed 15,000 adults from across the United States for more than 25 years. They were ages 45 to 66 at the start of the study. Biological aging was measured through 15 health markers that revealed a picture of how well a person's heart, lungs, metabolism, kidneys, and immune system were functioning.

The body needs water for every single thing it does, including pumping blood and nutrients to the brain and the rest of the body, so staying hydrated is essential. Good hydration supports brain performance, heart health, energy levels, healthy digestion, the body's natural detoxification systems, better temperature regulation, and decreased joint pain and headaches. We lose fluid all day through normal activities like breathing, urinating, bowel movements, and sweating. When the body is as little as 1 to 2 percent dehydrated, it can affect our memory, mood, concentration, and reaction time.

Unfortunately, a few things make it more challenging for older adults to stay hydrated. One, the thirst reflex goes down as we age into our sixties and beyond, which makes it easier for dehydration to silently sneak up on us. Two, with less muscle mass (which holds a lot of water), the older adult often has less overall fluid in the body. Three, there are many common medications older adults may take that create fluid loss. But by building healthy hydration habits, staying hydrated can be simple.

Signs You Are Dehydrated

- Dark urine
- Frequent but small amount of urine
- Dry mouth or coated tongue
- Constipation or small and hard stools
- Possibly due to dehydration: dry skin, frequent urinary tract infection, headache, confusion, dizziness or lightheadedness after standing up, fast heart rate, dry eyes

MIND Diet At-a-Glance

This is a simple and handy reference sheet for you to come back to or keep with you to remember what to eat (and limit) on the MIND diet.

What to Eat

Use this to check off weekly intake of MIND diet foods. Optional: note the day of the week in the blank box instead of a check mark. Each blank box is a serving. A separate chart is provided for whole grains since they are recommended three times a day.

- **Every day:** Three servings of whole grains, a serving of vegetables, olive oil, a glass of wine (5 ounces)
- **Most days:** Leafy green vegetables (6 times per week), nuts (5 times per week)
- **Every other day:** Beans (4 times per week)
- **Twice a week:** Berries, poultry
- **Once a week:** Seafood

WEEKLY TRACKER

LEAFY GREENS	OTHER VEGETABLES	NUTS	BEANS	BERRIES	

DAILY WHOLE GRAINS TRACKER

Sun	Mon	Tues	Wed	

WEEKLY TRACKER

	LEAN POULTRY	SEAFOOD	OLIVE OIL	5 OUNCES WINE (OPTIONAL)

DAILY WHOLE GRAINS TRACKER

	Thurs	Fri	Sat

What to Limit

These trackers will help keep you in line with the MIND diet recommendations. Place a check mark in one blank box for every time you ate these foods. Or, if you prefer, use the blank space to note the dates you had these foods and/or what you ate. The trackers have enough space to allow for the maximum allowance of these foods. Try to stay within these guidelines.

- **Less than one tablespoon per day:** Butter and stick margarine
- **No more than four times per week:** Pastries and sweets
- **No more than three times per week:** Red meat
- **No more than one serving every two weeks:** Whole-fat cheese, fried fast food

WEEKLY TRACKER: FOODS TO LIMIT

BUTTER AND STICK MARGARINE (< 1 TBSP)	PASTRIES & SWEETS	RED MEAT

WHOLE-FAT CHEESE	FRIED FAST FOOD

A Dash of Common Sense

Nourishing the body with good nutrition is about the big picture. It is never about single foods or single nutrients. It's about what they add up to and how they work together. This is why nutrition experts promote healthy eating *patterns* with a balance and variety of many healthy foods. The whole is more important than any parts on their own. While this makes healthy eating a more complex endeavor (some would say more interesting too), it is fundamental to good nutrition. There are a few "rules of thumb" that are fundamental to nutrition that are important to evaluating any diet advice.

There's More Than One Road to Health

The MIND diet is only one approach to healthful eating. For those most concerned about brain health, the MIND diet may do more good than not, and because the diet is based on the Mediterranean and DASH diets, there are many good reasons to follow this eating pattern for heart health and general well-being. Remember, though, that there are other healthy eating patterns, including culturally diverse eating patterns that promote heart health and longevity from around the world.

Sometimes More Isn't Better

A well-established rule in nutrition is that nutrients (and of course the foods that supply them) affect human health in a way that is not linear, which means that more of a good thing isn't always better. Sometimes it's just more, and other times, it's toxic. Instead, it's helpful to think of the way nutrients affect the body's functions as a bell curve. The body can function optimally within a fairly wide range of intake levels, but very low levels lead to deficiencies, and very high intakes lead to toxicity. Taking in nutrients at the low or high extremes can interrupt the body's ability to stay healthy, and can even lead to death.

Upgrades Are Essential

Another general rule is that healthy foods must replace unhealthy foods. To add nutritious foods to the diet and keep eating the harmful ones is a step in the right direction, but isn't enough. Similarly, eating healthy foods prepared in unhealthy ways (e.g., frying) doesn't confer the same benefits and can even negate them.

The Best Weight-Loss Diet

Any healthy diet, if followed with the concepts of balance, variety, and portions in mind, should also be ideal for weight management, even when they are not specifically designed for it. The best diet is the one that works for you.

Research-Based Cultural Adaptations of the MIND Diet

Chinese MIND Diet

- Whole grains, 250–400 g/day
- Fresh vegetables, 6x/week
- Mushroom or algae, 4x/week
- Fresh fruit, 6x/week

- Vegetable oil
- Fish, 1x/week
- Soybeans, 4x/week
- Nuts 5x/week

- Garlic, 4x/week
- Green tea, almost every day
- Pastries/sweets < 1x/month

Korean MIND Diet

- Vegetables, 6x/week
- Nuts, 6x/week
- Whole grains, 6x/week
- Perilla oil or powder, 6x/ week
- Milk or fermented milk, 6x/ week
- Water, 6x/week
- Legumes, 3x/week
- Fruits, 3x/week

- Berries, 3x/week
- Tomatoes, 3x/week
- Fish, 1x/week
- Poultry, 1x/week
- Social interaction, 1x/week 30+ min
- Physical activity, 1x/week 30+min
- No alcohol

Frequently Asked Questions

In the years since the first edition of this book came out in 2016, a lot of questions have come up from people who want to get specific on how to follow the MIND diet. There's no question too small or too basic. Here are answers to some of the top questions about the MIND diet.

What does the MIND diet stand for?

The MIND diet is an acronym for the Mediterranean-Dietary Approaches to Stop Hypertension (DASH) Intervention for Neuro-degenerative Delay diet. It is based on the Mediterranean and DASH diets, known for being heart-healthy, then optimized for brain health.

What foods are on the MIND diet?

The MIND includes 10 types of foods to eat more of: leafy green vegetables, more vegetables, nuts, beans, berries, lean poultry, fish, whole grains, olive oil, and moderate wine intake. It limits (but does not eliminate) intake of five types of food: red meat, butter, full-fat cheese, fried fast food, and pastries and sweets.

Can you eat eggs on the MIND diet?

Yes. In fact, eggs are an important source of brain-supportive nutrients, including choline and a carotenoid called lutein.

Can you drink coffee on the MIND diet?

Yes. The caffeine and antioxidants in coffee may be brain protective. A 2023 review paper by Porro et al. notes that caffeine lowers the risk of Alzheimer's disease, according to observational studies. Green and black teas are additional options for beverages that offer caffeine plus antioxidants.

Is peanut butter on the MIND diet?

Since peanuts are nutritionally similar to nuts, and technically a legume (which puts them in the same family of foods as beans), peanuts and peanut butter can definitely be part of the MIND diet. Peanuts are a good source of folate and vitamin E, two nutrients that are especially important for brain health. Check the label and look for peanut butter with minimal added sugars (< 2 g/serving) and salt (sodium < 150 mg/serving).

What cheese can I eat on the MIND diet?

You can enjoy a serving (1 ounce) of any cheese you like one to two times per month. The MIND diet doesn't eliminate any foods, though it does recommend limiting full-fat cheese intake to less than 1 ounce per week in order to minimize saturated fat intake. Cheeses that are relatively lower in saturated fat are queso fresco, part-skim ricotta, mozzarella, cottage cheese, soft goat cheese, feta, Neufchatel, camembert, Swiss, and parmesan, which all have less than 5 grams of saturated fat per serving. You may also opt for reduced fat cheese if you enjoy it.

Is oatmeal on the MIND diet?

Yes, because oatmeal is a whole grain. Steel cut oats offer a nice texture as a porridge, and rolled "traditional" oats can be eaten raw, so they work well in overnight oats and no-bake granola snacks.

Are potatoes OK on the MIND diet?

Yes, because potatoes are a vegetable. They provide potassium, vitamin C, and even some fiber and plant protein. They are delicious in stews, potato pancakes, or roasted with olive oil. Like all foods, it depends on how it's prepared. As a common fried fast food, French fries are not the healthiest way to enjoy potatoes. The MIND diet limits fried fast foods to one to two times per month.

Can you eat popcorn on the MIND diet?

Yes, because popcorn is a whole grain. Freshly popped popcorn smells so good and tastes great tossed with olive oil, a little salt, and herbs. Keep in mind that adding butter, cheese, or sugar will put popcorn into the "foods to limit" category, but not because of the popcorn itself.

Can you lose weight with the MIND diet?

The MIND diet is designed for brain health, not weight loss. However, the 2023 MIND diet trial had modest calorie-reduction built in and found that people lost 5.5 percent body weight and were able to keep it off for the duration of the three-year study while following the MIND diet. The study had higher-than-average retention rates, suggesting that the MIND diet was easy to stick to, perhaps because it's less restrictive than many other eating plans. In addition, if following the MIND diet means shifting away from the Standard American Diet (characterized by high calorie but low nutrition foods), it's reasonable to think this will naturally lead to some weight loss.

Is shrimp on the MIND diet?

Yes, shrimp can fit in the MIND diet. Shrimp offers lean protein and is a popular seafood choice in the United States. A 3-ounce serving of shrimp is high in the antioxidant selenium and vitamin B12. Though it is a very low-fat food with about half a gram of total fat per serving, the small amount of fat includes about 240 milligrams of omega-3s. It can also be a starter seafood before choosing fish with higher levels of omega-3s (500+ milligrams/serving), such as anchovies, oysters, salmon, sardines, tuna, barramundi, mussels, sea bass, and trout.

Are sweet potatoes on the MIND diet?

Yes, because sweet potatoes are a vegetable. They are high in fiber for gut health, antioxidants such as vitamin A and vitamin C, vitamin B6 to lower homocysteine (which is linked to dementia), and potassium, known for lowering blood pressure. They are most commonly a deep orange color, but purple flesh potatoes are also delicious, sweet, and nutritious.

Are avocados allowed on the MIND diet?

Yes, as a source of healthy fats and carotenoids like lutein, avocados are a great choice to eat while following the MIND diet. A 2021 review of 19 clinical trials by Dreher et al. found that Hass avocados improve cognitive function, especially executive function, in older adults as well as young to middle-age overweight and obese adults.

Is honey allowed on the MIND diet?

Yes, in modest amounts. Honey is a source of sugar that also provides some polyphenols, which gives it a nutritional edge over refined white sugar. Enjoyed in true moderation, any source of sugar can fit into a balanced diet. That said, sweeteners such as honey and maple syrup may be good choices for those who want less processed sources of sweetness. Date paste and prune puree are additional options.

Is Greek yogurt on the MIND diet?

There's no restriction on yogurt on the MIND diet—whether it's regular yogurt or a strained yogurt such as Greek yogurt or Icelandic skyr. The MIND diet aims to keep saturated fat low, so non-fat, low-fat, or reduced-fat yogurts are the most aligned with the MIND diet recommendations.

What fruits are allowed on the MIND diet?

All fruit is allowed on the MIND diet. Berries are the only fruit specifically recommended on the MIND diet, but there are no restrictions on other fruit. In fact, when the MIND diet has been adapted to non-Western cultures, eating a variety of fruit is highly encouraged.

Can you have almond milk on the MIND diet?

Yes, almond milk provides some of the nutrients from almonds, which are included in the MIND diet. Look for almond milk that is unsweetened. If almond milk is replacing animal milk or another plant milk, you may be gaining some nutrients but missing others. Just ensure that you are getting the nutrients you'll be missing out on from other foods.

Is hummus good for the brain?

Two of the main ingredients in hummus are chickpeas (beans) and olive oil, two of the recommended foods to eat on the MIND diet. You can feel good about enjoying hummus, especially if it acts as a carrier food to encourage you to eat more vegetables and whole grains, for example.

Is dark chocolate a part of the MIND diet?

Dark chocolate is not a part of the MIND diet, but it is a source of polyphenols that may help with inflammation, and bioactives that may improve brain function (and heart health) by increasing blood flow. A 2021 systematic review by Martin et al. found that regular intake of cocoa flavanols from chocolate improved cognitive performance in young adults. A 2021 systematic review by Tan et al. indicates that research among older adults is ongoing, with some mixed results.

Do I need to drink wine to benefit from the MIND diet?

The MIND diet includes a glass of wine a day, no more, no less, but you can reach therapeutic levels of the MIND diet without it, which is important since drinking alcohol isn't right for everyone. The wine component of the MIND diet has always been about finding a sweet spot for how much, if at all. At the end of the day, it's a matter of personal choice, perhaps informed by a discussion with your dietitian and care team. If you do choose to drink wine, keep it to one 5-ounce glass a day.

How does the MIND diet differ from the Mediterranean diet?

In general, the MIND diet is simpler and more permissive. Compared to the Mediterranean diet, the MIND diet has lower minimums for whole grains, potatoes, fish, and poultry. The vegetable minimum is lower, but it's more specific (leafy greens); same for fruit (berries). There is less dairy, with specific limits on butter and cheese. There's also a specific limit on fried fast food not specified on the Mediterranean diet. There are more nuts and beans and a greater allowance for red meat on the MIND diet. However, what they have in common is the central role of olive oil as the main dietary fat, and wine in moderation.

Is the MIND diet effective for preserving cognitive function?

Observational data suggest the MIND diet can reduce the risk of Alzheimer's disease by up to 53 percent and slow down biological aging in the brain by 7.5 years. The best clinical trial on the MIND diet found that it preserved cognitive function, but so did the control diet. Both diets reached therapeutic levels of the MIND diet (scores of 8.5 and above).

How do I get enough protein on the MIND diet?

The MIND diet includes a variety of protein sources from plants and animals to meet protein needs. Keep in mind that recommended foods are generally minimums (except wine), so meals can be adjusted to meet your protein needs. Protein foods associated with the MIND diet include beans, nuts, seafood, and lean poultry. Smaller amounts of protein are provided from fruit, vegetables, and whole grains, which contribute to overall daily protein intake.

Can you eat grits on the MIND diet?

Whole grain grits are a good option to enjoy on the MIND diet. For example, stone-ground grits include the entire kernel, including the germ and hull. Store them in the freezer to last longer. Quick or regular grits are a refined grain with the hull and germ removed. As a refined grain, it's better to enjoy these in moderation. There's no specific limit on refined grains with the MIND diet, but with an emphasis on whole grains, there is less room for them.

What can you substitute for butter on the MIND diet?

Olive oil is delicious and can be buttery and smooth or peppery when the polyphenols tickle the back of your throat. Either way, olive oil provides an indulgent mouthfeel, making it a good substitute for butter.

Can the MIND diet help my brain become more resilient?

Yes, research suggests the MIND diet has a role in building brain resilience. Research published in 2021[41] found that despite physical signs of Alzheimer's on the brain, people who closely followed the MIND diet had better cognitive function and slower cognitive decline than those with lower MIND diet scores. A similar phenomenon was seen in the brains of people who regularly ate seafood. Some seafood can be a source of mercury, a known neurotoxin, so it wasn't surprising that their brains had higher levels of mercury. But it was surprising that these same brains had lower signs of Alzheimer's. What these studies point to is that what we eat builds up our cognitive resilience, or the brain's ability to overcome challenges. The brain is challenged

---

41 K. Dhana et al., "Common Brain Pathologies and Cognition in Community-Dwelling Older Adults," *Journal of Alzheimer's Disease* 83, no. 2 (2021): 683–692, doi: 10.3233/JAD-210107.

by air pollution, stress, and more, so the more we can mitigate their effects, the better.

How does menopause affect the risk for Alzheimer's?

After older age, being female is the next major risk factor for developing Alzheimer's disease. Two out of every three Alzheimer's patients are women. Of these women, 60 percent are post-menopausal. This is an active area of study that has historically been under-studied, but what we do know is that estrogen seems to protect the brain against neurodegenerative diseases like Alzheimer's disease. Researchers think menopause-related drops in estrogen are setting the stage for brain changes in midlife that increase the risk for Alzheimer's. It is now widely accepted that our health in midlife affects our late-life brain health, and that there are 15 to 20 years when brain changes are happening silently before signs of Alzheimer's are clinically detectable.[42] It's never too late or too early for women to eat well for brain health, but midlife may be an especially important time to cement healthy habits.

Can the MIND diet protect cognition in post-menopausal women?

A small three-month study in 68 post-menopausal women ages 60 to 75 found that a combination of following the MIND diet and walking three times a week led to improved cognitive function.[43] The women walked on a treadmill for 40 minutes at 60 to 70 percent maximum effort with a 10-minute warm-up and 10-minute cooldown for a total of 60 active minutes.

In addition, several studies show that women (and men) following the MIND diet in midlife have better cardiovascular health and a

---

42 Sperling et al., "The Evolution of Preclinical Alzheimer's Disease," *Neuron* 84, no. 3 (2014): 608–622, doi: 10.1016/j.neuron.2014.10.038.

43 Elsayed et al., "Aerobic Exercise with Mediterranean-DASH Intervention for Neurodegenerative Delay Diet Promotes Brain Cells' Longevity despite Sex Hormone Deficiency in Postmenopausal Women," *Oxidative Medicine and Cellular Longevity*, 2022: 4146742, doi: 10.1155/2022/4146742.

reduced risk of cognitive decline and Alzheimer's disease compared to those with lower MIND diet scores.

Can the MIND diet help with brain fog?

The MIND diet is specifically designed to alleviate many of the symptoms related to brain fog. First, it's useful to understand that "brain fog" is a nonclinical term used by patients and the healthcare community to describe a range of cognitive complaints. It could refer to any combination of difficulty focusing, short-term memory loss, having a hard time switching tasks, slower processing time, slower working memory, or challenges with sound decision-making. It could be a response to poor sleep, poor nutrition, medications, or chronic neuroinflammation.

Studies show high-polyphenol foods such as dark green leafy vegetables, wild blueberries, walnuts, and olive oil improve cognitive function. Rich sources of dietary fiber, such as beans, nuts, and some dried fruit support a robust microbiome that in turn supports brain health. Poor microbiome health leads to systemic inflammation that can weaken the blood-brain barrier.

Anti-inflammatory omega-3s in foods such as fatty fish, flaxseed, and walnuts also support optimal brain function by maintaining the integrity of neuronal cell membranes. The brain is one of the body's most metabolically active organs, so it has a high need for antioxidants and anti-inflammatory molecules.

Eating patterns high in added sugars and saturated fats and low in polyphenols and dietary fiber are associated with greater rates of anxiety, depression, and cognition issues, which are hallmarks of brain fog. Therefore, foods to limit include sugary foods and drinks, fried foods, some cuts of red meat, hard cheeses, and solid cooking fats like butter and coconut oil. Keep in mind that limit doesn't mean eliminate, and that it's all about balance. If you enjoy these foods, they should be in smaller amounts compared to an overall eating pattern dominated by wholesome choices such as vegetables, fruits, whole grains, lean proteins, seafood, nuts, beans, and mostly unsaturated oils.

Overall, the MIND diet encourages eating the foods that will help clear brain fog and reduces the foods most likely to exacerbate it.

What are the most common types of brain fog?

- **Menopause brain fog:** Brain fog is a reliably documented symptom of menopause and is described as the cognitive symptoms women experience around menopause, including memory and attention problems. It may present as difficulty remembering words or names, having a hard time maintaining a train of thought, being easily distracted, or forgetting why you came into a specific room. The decline in estrogen, poor sleep quality, and low mood common around menopause may be behind memory and cognition changes, though cause-and-effect is not yet proven.

- **COVID-19 brain fog:** Cognitive impairment is one of the most common complaints of post-COVID syndrome, affecting about a third of patients by some estimates, and shows up after both severe and mild cases. This kind of brain fog often affects attention, executive function, and memory. The causes are not yet well understood, though researchers hypothesize it could be from a lack of oxygen, damage to blood vessels, or chronic inflammation.

- **ADHD brain fog:** Symptoms of ADHD and brain fog are similar, and one published case study suggests the symptoms of a post-COVID patient with brain fog can be successfully treated as an ADHD-like condition. This was only one case study, so it's important to replicate these findings with stronger research.

- **Pregnancy brain fog:** So-called "pregnancy brain" is not well-documented in research, but there is enough to show that working memory takes a hit during pregnancy. Cognitive changes are likely due to the impact of hormonal changes to the brain. Women with fibromyalgia often experience more severe symptoms during the third and fourth trimesters of pregnancy, including brain fog.

Should I be taking an omega-3 supplement for brain health?

The Global Council on Brain Health and the Alzheimer's Association agree that there is not yet enough evidence to recommend supplements in general for brain health at this time. But we know omega-3s are good for the brain, so what about omega-3 supplements? The choice to take supplements should be made in partnership with your healthcare team to address your individual needs. Supplements may fill gaps not met by the diet, but should not replace a healthy balanced diet.

Research on omega-3 supplements can be confusing when it doesn't all say the same thing. There are a few reasons for this.

1. **Mixed outcomes may be the result of different methods.** One of the most common issues is when baseline levels of the nutrient being studied aren't measured. For example, a 2023 review paper by Hersant et al. found no compelling evidence to take omega-3 supplements for memory. On the other hand, when a population is low in omega-3s and at risk for cognitive decline, we often see research-backed benefits for omega-3 supplementation.

2. **Supplements may not work the same way in all people.** We know women and people of color are underrepresented in research, so the American Heart Association reviewed the available evidence for fish and omega-3s in these populations in a 2024 review paper by Welty et al. They found that lifelong non-fried fatty fish intake was associated with preventing cognitive decline. In randomized controlled trials, women saw cognition benefits from omega-3 EPA and DHA supplementation, where DHA seemed more

helpful than EPA, and that supplementation works better if it's started before cognitive decline starts. For cardiovascular disease prevention, men and women, including Black and Asian populations, benefited from eating fish and EPA and DHA supplementation.

If you do decide taking an omega-3 supplement is right for you, know that it will be better absorbed if taken at the same time you eat fatty foods. Therefore, consider taking it with foods that provide healthy fats, including omega-3s, such as fatty fish, perilla oil, walnuts, chia seeds, and flaxseed.

What are the most effective supplements for memory and cognition?

As mentioned, the Global Council on Brain Health and the Alzheimer's Association agree that there is not yet enough evidence to recommend supplements in general for brain health at this time. Many supplements make memory and cognition claims, but they don't all have solid science behind them. In general, if you are low in essential nutrients important for brain function, such as B-vitamins, vitamin D, or vitamin E, then a supplement should help. If there is no nutrient gap to fill, you don't need a supplement.

That said, in four recent large randomized clinical trials published in 2023 and 2024, a humble daily multivitamin improved cognitive outcomes.[44,45,46,47] A 2024 review paper by Hersant et al. suggests there is some evidence that ashwagandha, choline, curcumin, ginger, lion's mane, polyphenols, phosphatidylserine, probiotics, and turmeric

44   Vyas et al., "Effect of Multivitamin-Mineral Supplementation versus Placebo on Cognitive Function," *American Journal of Clinical Nutrition* 119, no. 3, (2024) 692–701.

45   Sachs et al., "Impact of Multivitamin-Mineral and Cocoa Extract on Incidence of Mild Cognitive Impairment and Dementia," *Alzheimer's & Dementia* 19, no. 11 (2023) 4863–4871.

46   Yeung et al., "Multivitamin Supplementation Improves Memory in Older Adults," *American Journal of Clinical Nutrition* 118, no. 1 (2023) 273–282.

47   Baker et al., "Effects of Coca Extract and a Multivitamin on Cognitive Function," *Alzheimer's & Dementia* 19, no. 4 (2023): 1308–1319.

may provide memory benefits. There are mixed results regarding the benefit of carnitine, gingko biloba, and huperzine A.

At the end of the day, the choice to supplement your diet is a personal one that can be discussed with your healthcare team, but there is no substitute for a healthy diet.

Are all processed foods bad for brain health?

No, not all processed foods are unhealthy. It's important to distinguish between ultra-processed and simply processed. Cooking food at home is a form of processing, for example, even though it's linked with healthier eating. In fact, many "processed" foods are very healthful. For example, canned beans, shelled nuts, whole grains, and frozen fruit are all technically "processed" before you buy them in the grocery store. Even some foods categorized as "ultra-processed" have benefits, such as soy milk.

Should I be worried about ultra-processed foods?

Yes and no. First, the processing is not the issue, but the fact that there is a high correlation between ultra-processing and unhealthful foods makes it a good shortcut for recommending which foods to cut. As noted in the previous question, some ultra-proceed foods are quite healthy. The problem is that most aren't, and so yes, there is reason to be wary.

Unhealthy ultra-processed foods increase the risk of dementia in a dose-response manner. That means the more you eat these foods, the greater your risk. People who eat too many ultra-processed foods (UPF) are 44 percent more likely to develop dementia according to 2024 research by Henney et al. that analyzed findings from 10 observational studies that examined 867,316 people. That's compared to people who ate a low amount of UPF. A study from 2022 by Hecht et al. found that high UPF diets also increased the risk of depression by 81 percent and the likelihood of more anxious days per month.

UPF tend to be calorie-rich and nutrient-poor, highly palatable, and convenient. Some of the most common ones are reconstituted meat products, packaged snacks, chips, breakfast cereals, cookies, cake, and breads. If some of your favorite foods were in that list, be comforted that there is still room to enjoy them. But it needs to be rebalanced. More than half (60 percent) of all calories come from UPF in the United States[48], even though it should be closer to a quarter of that (15 percent). And of course, the devil is in the details. Not every single food in those categories are UPF, and not every UPF is unhealthy. Your best bet is to primarily choose whole foods; for everything else, take a close look at the nutrition label to make informed choices.

What are ultra-processed foods?

Ultra-processed foods (UPF) are, as the name suggests, highly processed. They are industrial formulations of foods that have undergone extensive transformation. For example, sugar-sweetened soft drinks, candy, and processed meat. They often contain added colors, flavors, and preservatives. Ultra-processed foods are often high in calories, added sugar, saturated fat, and salt, but low in protein, fiber, vitamins, minerals, and phytochemicals.

It's a technical term used in research and refers to one of four levels of processing within the NOVA classification system, the most widely used and internationally accepted system of organizing foods by level of processing. Though it is meant for researchers, it has reached media and consumers, and can cause confusion.

It's important to know that the processing itself is not the issue (consider that all foods in the grocery store have undergone some kind of processing to arrive at the store). Even the hallmark ingredients in UPF, such as protein isolates, are not the issue. The issue is that most of what we eat qualifies as a UPF, and this is displacing fruits, vegetables, and home-made meals that offer better nutrition.

---

48   Hecht et al., "Cross-Sectional Examination of Ultra-processed Food Consumption and Adverse Mental Health Symptoms," *Public Health Nutrition* 25, no. 11 (2022): 3225–3234, doi: 10.1017/S1368980022001586.

This is why research shows a connection between eating too many UPF and poor health outcomes. Seventy percent[49] of all packaged foods qualify as UPF in the United States. Studies have found an association between high intakes of UPF and dementia as well as poor mental health.[50]

Bottomline: It's not about completely eliminating these foods if you enjoy them, but it is about rebalancing overall intake so that they take up a smaller share of your daily calories.

How does the MIND diet compare to other diets for brain health?

Several studies compare the MIND diet to its component diets, the Mediterranean diet and the Dietary Approaches to Stop Hypertension (DASH) diet. For the most part, the MIND diet performs as well or better than either of these when it comes to slowing cognitive decline and reducing the risk of Alzheimer's. What's more, the MIND diet is often protective when followed at both high and moderate levels, whereas brain-protective effects often disappear for the Mediterranean and DASH diets when only followed moderately.

The MIND diet has also been compared to ketogenic, modified Mediterranean-ketogenic, Seventh-Day Adventist, and anti-inflammatory diets. Of these, the Mediterranean-ketogenic diet may be the least familiar. It keeps the fruit and vegetable intake of the Mediterranean diet, but restricts overall carbohydrates, and increases the amount of fat and protein. For those not familiar, the Seventh-Day Adventist diet is a plant-forward diet followed by members of the Seventh-day Adventist Church since its formation in the mid-19th century. Many are vegan, while others include small amounts of

---

49 Hecht et al., "Cross-Sectional Examination of Ultra-processed Food Consumption."

50 Hecht et al., "Cross-Sectional Examination of Ultra-processed Food Consumption"; Henney et al., "High Intake of Ultra-processed Food Is Associated with Dementia in Adults," *Journal of Neurology*, 271, no. 1 (2024): 198–210, doi: 10.1007/s00415-023-12033-1.

animal foods. They're also encouraged to avoid caffeine, sweeteners, refined foods, alcohol, smoking, and drugs.

To some extent, all of these dietary patterns have been associated with better cognitive outcomes. The most consistent evidence is for the MIND and Mediterranean diets. There is limited research on Seventh-Day Adventist or the anti-inflammatory diet, though the positive results make sense since they are plant-based diets like MIND and Mediterranean diets. In small trials, ketogenic and modified Mediterranean-ketogenic diets have improved cognitive function. However, researchers note that maintaining a ketogenic diet may be challenging for older adults due to side effects and ability to get all the nutrients needed.

What's the difference between dementia and Alzheimer's disease?

Alzheimer's disease is the most common cause of dementia, but not all dementia is caused by Alzheimer's disease. Dementia is not a specific disease. Instead it is the name for a group of symptoms caused by disorders that affect the brain, including Alzheimer's disease and stroke. The most common symptom is memory loss. It is not a normal part of aging. Alzheimer's disease is a disease that causes large numbers of nerve cells in the brain to die, commonly marked by memory loss plus cognitive decline in one or more other areas such as language skills, reasoning, attention, or visual perception.

GLOSSARY

Alzheimer's disease

Alzheimer's disease is a disease that causes large numbers of nerve cells in the brain to die, commonly marked by memory loss plus cognitive decline in one or more other areas such as language skills, reasoning, attention, or visual perception. It is the most common cause of dementia.

Apolipoprotein E genotyping

Apolipoprotein E (APOE) genotyping is a secondary lab test that may help diagnose late-onset Alzheimer's disease in adults who show symptoms. If a person with dementia also has APOE-e4, it may be more likely that dementia is due to Alzheimer's disease, but it cannot prove it. In fact, there are no definitive diagnostic tests for Alzheimer's disease during life. This test is not appropriate for screening people without symptoms, and some people with APOE-e4 will never develop Alzheimer's disease.

Beta-amyloid

The accumulation of beta-amyloid proteins form plaques that eventually disrupt nerve cell function, leading to the death of the affected brain cells, which is believed to be a culprit in Alzheimer's disease.

Cognition

Cognition is the ability to think, learn, and remember. It is the basis for how we reason, judge, concentrate, plan, and organize.

Cognitive decline

Cognitive decline describes the loss of cognitive abilities that occurs as a normal part of the aging process. It is differentiated from mild cognitive impairment, Alzheimer's disease, and dementia, which are all abnormal conditions.

Cognitive reserve

Cognitive reserve is related to cognitive resilience and describes the set of tools and resources a brain has available, such as education, cognitive performance, and career attainment, to actively compensate for brain pathologies. It is a concept used to estimate cognitive resilience. A person with a strong cognitive reserve is more likely to show greater cognitive resilience.

Cognitive resilience

Cognitive resilience is the brain's ability to cope, adapt, and perform despite brain changes related to mild cognitive decline or Alzheimer's, Parkinson's disease, multiple sclerosis, stroke, stress, or surgery. A person who shows more cognitive resilience likely has a deeper cognitive reserve to pull from.

Dementia

Dementia is not a specific disease. Instead it is the name for a group of symptoms caused by disorders that affect the brain, including Alzheimer's disease and stroke. The most common symptom is memory loss. It is not a normal part of aging.

Dietary Approaches to Stop Hypertension (DASH)

Dietary Approaches to Stop Hypertension (DASH) is a healthy eating pattern developed for research on how diet can reduce blood pressure. It emphasizes eating plenty of vegetables, fruits, and whole grains. It also includes fat-free or low-fat dairy, plus fish, poultry, beans, nuts, and vegetable oils. It discourages foods that are high in saturated fat, such as fatty meats, full-fat dairy products, and tropical oils such as coconut, palm kernel, and palm oils. It also limits added sugar.

Episodic memory

Episodic memory is our personal memory of events at a certain time and place. These memories are specific to each of us and can have an emotional aspect.

Five cognitive domains

The five cognitive domains are: episodic memory, working memory, semantic memory, visuospatial ability, and perceptual speed.

Inflammaging

Inflammaging is the increase in pro-inflammatory markers in the blood and tissues that rise with advancing age to create mild chronic inflammation, which is a risk factor for accelerated aging and susceptibility to all diseases. It is associated with cognitive disability and dementia as well as physical disability, frailty, premature death, cardiovascular diseases, type 2 diabetes, chronic kidney disease, cancers, depression, osteoporosis, sarcopenia, and anemia.

Mediterranean Diet

The Mediterranean Diet is a healthy eating pattern based on traditional foods and beverages from the countries bordering the Mediterranean Sea. Despite variations in the specifics of the foods due to cultural and social differences, key components are fruits, vegetables, whole grains, olive oil, beans, nuts, legumes, seeds, herbs, spices, fish and seafood, with some, but less, poultry, eggs, cheese, yogurt, and occasional wine.

Memory and Aging Project (MAP)

Memory and Aging Project (MAP) is a research study conducted by Rush University Medical Center in Chicago, IL, supported by the National Institute on Aging. The study seeks to better understand, treat, and, hopefully, prevent the problems with memory, mobility, and strength associated with abnormal aging.

Mild cognitive impairment (MCI)

Mild cognitive impairment is also referred to as MCI. It is a medical condition that causes people to have more memory problems than other people their age. The signs of MCI are not as severe as those of Alzheimer's disease.

MIND diet

The MIND diet is an acronym for the Mediterranean-Dietary Approaches to Stop Hypertension (DASH) Intervention for Neurodegenerative Delay diet. It is based on the Mediterranean and DASH diets, known for being heart-healthy, then optimized for brain health. It includes 10 types of foods to eat more of: leafy green vegetables, additional vegetables, nuts, beans, berries, lean poultry, fish, whole grains, olive oil, and moderate wine intake. It limits (but does not eliminate) intake of five types of food: red meat, butter, full-fat cheese, fried fast food, and pastries and sweets.

Neuron

Neurons commonly refer to brain cells, though they technically include any nerve impulse–conducting cell in the nervous system, including nerve, brain, or spinal column cells.

Nurses' Health Study

The Nurses' Health Studies (NHS) are among the largest and longest running investigations of factors that influence women's health. Started in 1976 and expanded in 1989, the information provided by the 238,000 dedicated nurse-participants has led to many new insights on health and disease. While the prevention of cancer is still a primary focus, the study has also produced landmark data on cardiovascular disease, diabetes, and many other conditions. Most importantly, these studies have shown that diet, physical activity, and other lifestyle factors can powerfully promote better health.

NHS is affiliated with Harvard Medical School, Harvard School of Public Health, Brigham and Women's Hospital, Dana Farber Cancer Institute, Children's Hospital of Boston, Beth Israel Deaconess Medical Center, and Channing Laboratory.

Perceptual speed

Perceptual speed is assessed by the speed of responding (usually using paper-and-pencil tests) with simple content in which everyone would be perfect if there were no time limits.

Semantic memory

Semantic memory refers to a kind of long-term memory that includes knowledge of facts, events, ideas, and concepts.

Subjective cognitive decline

Subjective cognitive decline (SCD) is a self-reported increase in confusion and memory loss over the past 12 months. It is a type of cognitive impairment. It is not a formal diagnosis, but may be an early symptom of dementia. In the US, it affects one in nine adults.

Tau tangles

Tau is a protein that helps form straight and strong microtubules that transport nutrients within brain neurons. When tau proteins collapse, they clump to each other and these are called tau tangles. Nutrients aren't transported and cells eventually die. Tau tangles are a hallmark of Alzheimer's disease.

Visuospatial memory

Visuospatial memory is the ability to understand the spatial relationship between objects. It helps the brain see something and/or its working parts, then understand and replicate it.

Working memory

Working memory is more commonly known as short-term memory, and describes the ability to hold and use information in the moment. For example, doing mental arithmetic.

RESOURCES & REFERENCES

Resources

MIND Diet News & Recipes

- MIND Diet Meals: minddietmeals.com
- @minddietmeals: instagram.com/minddietmeals

Engage Your Brain

- Center for Brain Health events: centerforbrainhealth.org/events
- Healthy Brain Resource Center: nccd.cdc.gove/DPH_HBRC
- Let's Talk Brain Health podcast: virtualbrainhealthcenter.com/podcast
- Staying Sharp online program: stayingsharp.aarp.org

Healthy Aging

- Administration on Aging: aoa.gov
- Healthy Aging Program: cdc.gov/aging
- National Institute on Aging: nia.nih.gov
- National Association of Area Agencies on Aging: n4a.org

Alzheimer's Disease

- Alzheimer's Association: alz.org
- Alzheimer's Disease Education and Referral Center: www.nia.nih.gov/health/alzheimers-and-dementia
- Family Caregiver Alliance: caregiver.org
- National Alliance for Caregiving: caregiving.org

Healthy Foods

- Academy of Nutrition and Dietetics: foodandnutrition.org
- The Bean Institute: beaninstitute.com
- California Almond Board: almonds.com
- California Olive Oil Council: cooc.com
- California Strawberries: californiastrawberries.com
- California Walnut Commission: walnuts.org
- Canned Food Alliance: mealtime.org
- Cranberry Institute: cranberryinstitute.org
- FDA Advice about eating fish: fda.gov/food/consumers/advice -about-eating-fish
- Fruits and Veggies More Matters: fruitsandveggies.org
- International Tree Nut Council Nutrition Research and Education Foundation: nuthealth.org
- Monterey Bay Aquarium Seafood Watch: seafoodwatch.org
- National Peanut Board: nationalpeanutboard.org
- Oldways Whole Grains Council: wholegrainscouncil.org
- Olive Wellness Institute: olivewellnessinstitute.org
- Red Raspberries: redrazz.org
- Seafood Nutrition Partnership: seafoodnutrition.org
- U.S. Highbush Blueberry Council: blueberry.org
- USDA MyPlate: choosemyplate.gov
- Wild Blueberry Association of North America: wildblueberries.com

Food Safety

- Federal Food Safety Gateway: foodsafety.gov
- Fight BAC!®: fightbac.org
- USDA Meat and Poultry Hotline: 1-888-MPHotline (1-888-674-6854) TTY: 1-800-256-7072. Hours: 10:00 a.m. to 4:00 p.m. Eastern time, Monday through Friday, in English and Spanish, or email: mphotline.fsis@usda.gov
- Visit "Ask Karen," FSIS's Web-based automated response system: fsis.usda.gov

References

MIND Diet

Agarwal, P., Y. Wang, A. S. Buchman, et al. "Dietary Patterns and Self-Reported Incident Disability in Older Adults." *The Journals of Gerontology. Series A, Biological Sciences and Medical Sciences.* 2019; 74 (8): 1331–1337. https://doi.org/10.1093/gerona/gly211.

Agarwal, P., Y. Wang. A. S. Buchman, et al. "MIND Diet Associated with Reduced Incidence and Delayed Progression of Parkinsonism" in Old Age." *The Journal of Nutrition, Health, and Aging.* 2018; 22: 1211–1215. doi: 10.1007/s12603-018-1094-5.

Arjmand, G., M. Abbas-Zadeh, M.Fardaei, et al. "The Effect of Short-Term Mediterranean-DASH Intervention for Neurodegenerative Delay (MIND) Diet on Hunger Hormones, Anthropometric Parameters, and Brain Structures in Middle-Aged Overweight and Obese Women: A Randomized Controlled Trial." *Iranian Journal of Medical Sciences.* 2022: 422–432. https://doi.org/10.30476/IJMS.2021.90829.2180.

Barkhordari, R., M. Namayandeh, M. Mirzaei, et al. "The Relation between MIND Diet with Psychological Disorders and Psychological Stress among Iranian Adults." *BMC Psychiatry.* 2022: 22 (1): 496. https://doi.org/10.1186/s12888-022-04128-2.

Barnes, L. L., K. Dhana, X. Liu, et al. "Trial of the MIND Diet for Prevention of Cognitive Decline in Older Persons." *The New England*

Journal of Medicine. 2023; 389 (7): 602–611. https://doi.org/10.1056/NEJ
Moa2302368.

Chan, R. S. M., B. W. M. Yu, J. Leung, et al. "How Dietary Patterns Are
Related to Inflammaging and Mortality in Community-Dwelling Older
Chinese Adults in Hong Kong—A Prospective Analysis." *The Journal of
Nutrition, Health, and Aging*. 2019: *23*(2): 181–194. https://doi.org
/10.1007/s12603-018-1143-0.

de la Monte S. M., J. R. Wands. "Alzheimer's Disease Is Type 3 Diabetes-
Evidence Reviewed." *J Diabetes Sci Technol*. 2008; 2(6): 1101–1113. doi:
10.1177/193229680800200619.

Dhana, K., O. H. Franco, E. M. Ritz, et al. "Healthy Lifestyle and Life
Expectancy with and without Alzheimer's Dementia: Population Based
Cohort Study." *BMJ (Clinical Research Ed.)*. 2022; *377* (e068390).
https://doi.org/10.1136/bmj-2021-068390.

Ferguson, C. C., S. E. Jung, J. C. Lawrence, et al. "A Mixed Methods
Exploration of the Impact of the COVID-19 Pandemic on Food-
Related Activities and Diet Quality in People with Parkinson Disease."
International Journal of Environmental Research and Public Health. 2022;
19(18): 11741. doi: 10.3390/ijerph191811741.

Fox, D. J., S. J. Park, and L. K. Mischley. "Comparison of Associations
between MIND and Mediterranean Diet Scores with Patient-Reported
Outcomes in Parkinson's Disease." *Nutrients*. 2022; 14(23): 5185. doi:
10.3390/nu14235185.

Gómez-Martínez, C., N. Babio, J. Júlvez, et al. "Impulsivity Is Longitu-
dinally Associated with Healthy and Unhealthy Dietary Patterns in
Individuals with Overweight or Obesity and Metabolic Syndrome within
the Framework of the PREDIMED-Plus Trial." *The International Journal
of Behavioral Nutrition and Physical Activity*. 2022; 19(1): 101. https://doi
.org/10.1186/s12966-022-01335-8.

Holthaus, T. A., S. Sethi, C. N. Cannavale, et al. "MIND Dietary Pattern
Adherence Is Inversely Associated with Visceral Adiposity and Features
of Metabolic Syndrome." *Nutrition Research (New York, N.Y.)*. 2023; 116:
69–79. https://doi.org/10.1016/j.nutres.2023.06.001.

Huang, X., S. Aihemaitijiang, C. Ye, et al. "Development of the cMIND
Diet and Its Association with Cognitive Impairment in Older Chinese
People." *The Journal of Nutrition, Health, and Aging*. 2022; 26(8):
760–770. https://doi.org/10.1007/s12603-022-1829-1.

Kang, E. Y., D. Kim, H. K. Kim, et al. "Modified Korean MIND Diet: A Nutritional Intervention for Improved Cognitive Function in Elderly Women through Mitochondrial Respiration, Inflammation Suppression, and Amino Acid Metabolism Regulation." *Molecular Nutrition & Food Research*. 2023; 67(20): 2300329. https://doi.org /10.1002/mnfr.202300329.

Kellar, D., and S. Craft. "Brain Insulin Resistance in Alzheimer's disease and Related Disorders: Mechanisms and Therapeutic Approaches." *The Lancet Neurology*. 2020; 19(9): 758–766. doi: 10.1016/S1474-4422(20): 30231-3.

Knight, E., T. Geetha, D. Burnett D, and J. R. Babu. "The Role of Diet and Dietary Patterns in Parkinson's Disease." *Nutrients*. 2022; 14(21): 4472. doi: 10.3390/nu14214472.

Lin, W., X. Zhou, and X. Liu. "Association of Adherence to the Chinese Version of the MIND Diet with Reduced Cognitive Decline in Older Chinese Individuals: Analysis of the Chinese Longitudinal Healthy Longevity Survey." *The Journal of Nutrition, Health, and Aging*. 2024; 28(2): 100024. https://doi.org/10.1016/j.jnha.2023.100024.

Metcalfe-Roach, A., A. C. Yu, E. Golz, et al. "MIND and Mediterranean Diets Associated with Later Onset of Parkinson's Disease." *Mov Disord*. 2021; 36(4): 977–984. doi: 10.1002/mds.28464.

Morris, M. C., C. C. Tangney, Y. Wang, et al. "MIND Diet Slows Cognitive Decline with Aging." *Alzheimer's & Dementia*. 2015; 11: 1015–1022.

Morris, M. C., C. C. Tangney, Y. Wang, et al. "MIND Diet Associated with Reduced Incidence of Alzheimer's Disease." *Alzheimer's & Dementia*. 2015; 11: 1007–1014.

Salari-Moghaddam, A., A. H. Keshteli, S. M. Mousavi, et al. "Adherence to the MIND Diet and Prevalence of Psychological Disorders in Adults." *Journal of Affective Disorders*. 2019; 256: 96–102. https://doi.org/10.1016 /j.jad.2019.05.056.

Song, Y., Z. Chang, K. Cui, et al. "The Value of the MIND Diet in the Primary and Secondary Prevention of Hypertension: A Cross-Sectional and Longitudinal Cohort Study from NHANES Analysis." *Frontiers in Nutrition*. 2023; 10: 1129667. https://doi.org/10.3389/fnut.2023.1129667.

Song, Y., Z. Chang, L. Jia, et al. "Better Adherence to the MIND Diet Is Associated with Lower Risk of All-Cause Death and Cardiovascular Death in Patients with Atherosclerotic Cardiovascular Disease or Stroke:

A Cohort Study from NHANES Analysis." *Food & Function*. 2023; 14(3): 1740–1749. https://doi.org/10.1039/d2fo03066g.

Song, Y., Z. Chang, C. Song, et al. "Association Between MIND Diet Adherence and Mortality: Insights from Diabetic and Non-Diabetic Cohorts." *Nutrition & Diabetes*. 2023; 13(1): 18. https://doi.org/10.1038/s41387-023-00247-1.

Talegawkar, S. A., Y. Jin, E. M. Simonsick, et al. "The Mediterranean-DASH Intervention for Neurodegenerative Delay (MIND) Diet Is Associated with Physical Function and Grip Strength in Older Men and Women." *The American Journal of Clinical Nutrition*. 2022; 115(3): 625–632. https://doi.org/10.1093/ajcn/nqab310.

Thomas, A., S. Lefèvre-Arbogast, C. Féart, et al. "Association of a MIND Diet with Brain Structure and Dementia in a French Population." *Journal of Prevention of Alzheimers Disease*. 2022; 9(4): 655–664. doi: 10.14283/jpad.2022.67.

Tison, S. E., J. M. Shikany, D. L. Long, et al. "Differences in the Association of Select Dietary Measures With Risk of Incident Type 2 Diabetes." *Diabetes Care*. 2022; 45(11): 2602–2610. https://doi.org/10.2337/dc22-0217.

Torabynasab, K., H. Shahinfar, S. Jazayeri, et al. "Adherence to the MIND Diet Is Inversely Associated with Odds and Severity of Anxiety Disorders: A Case-Control Study." *BMC Psychiatry*. 2023; 23(1): 330. https://doi.org/10.1186/s12888-023-04776-y.

Van Soest, A. P., S. Beers, O. van de Rest, et al. "The Mediterranean-Dietary Approaches to Stop Hypertension Intervention for Neurodegenerative Delay Diet for the Aging Brain: A Systematic Review." *Advances in Nutrition (Bethesda, Md.)*. 2024; 100184. https://doi.org/10.1016/j.advnut.2024.100184.

Walker, M. E., A. A. O'Donnell, J. J. Himali, et al. "Associations of the Mediterranean-Dietary Approaches to Stop Hypertension Intervention for Neurodegenerative Delay Diet with Cardiac Remodelling in the Community: The Framingham Heart Study." *The British Journal of Nutrition*. 2021; 126(12): 1888–1896. https://doi.org/10.1017/S0007114521000660.

Wang, Y., C. Haskell-Ramsay, J. L. Gallegos, et al. "Effects of Chronic Consumption of Specific Fruit (Berries, Cherries, and Citrus) on Cognitive Health: A Systematic Review and Meta-Analysis of

Randomised Controlled Trials." *European Journal of Clinical Nutrition.* 2023; 77(1): 7–22. https://doi.org/10.1038/s41430-022-01138-x.

Yau, K.-Y., P.-S. Law, and C.-N. Wong. "Cardiac and Mental Benefits of Mediterranean-DASH Intervention for Neurodegenerative Delay (MIND) Diet Plus Forest Bathing (FB) versus MIND Diet among Older Chinese Adults: A Randomized Controlled Pilot Study." *International Journal of Environmental Research and Public Health.* 2022; 19(22): 14665. https://doi.org/10.3390/ijerph192214665.

Vegetables and Leafy Greens

Chen, X., Y. Huang, and H. G. Cheng. "Lower Intake of Vegetables and Legumes Associated with Cognitive Decline Among Illiterate Elderly Chinese: A 3-Year Cohort Study." *The Journal of Nutrition, Health, and Aging.* 2012; 16: 549–552.

Haskell-Ramsay, C. F., and S. Docherty. "Role of Fruit and Vegetables in Sustaining Healthy Cognitive Function: Evidence and Issues." *Proceedings of the Nutrition Society.* 2023; 82(3): 305–314. https://doi .org/10.1017/S0029665123002999.

Kang, J. H., A. Ascherio, and F. Grodstein. "Fruit and Vegetable Consumption and Cognitive Decline in Aging Women." *Annals of Neurology.* 2005; 57: 713–720.

Morris, M. C., D. A. Evans, C. C. Tangney, et al. "Associations of Vegetable and Fruit Consumption with Age-Related Cognitive Change." *Neurology.* 2006; 67: 1370–1376.

Morris, M. C., C. C. Tangney, D. A. Evans, et al. "Fruit and Vegetable Consumption and Change in Cognitive Function in a Large Biracial Population." *American Journal of Epidemiology.* 2004; 166 (suppl): S63.

Morris, M. C., Y. Wang, L. L., et al. "Nutrients and Bioactives in Green Leafy Vegetables and Cognitive Decline." *Neurology.* 2018; 90(3): e214–e222. https://doi.org/10.1212/WNL.0000000000004815.

Nooyens, A. C., H. B. Bueno-de-Mesquita, M. P. van Boxtel, et al. "Fruit and Vegetable Intake and Cognitive Decline in Middle-Aged Men and Women: The Doetinchem Cohort Study." *British Journal of Nutrition.* 2011; 106: 752–761.

Whole Grains

Hardy, K., J. Brand-Miller, et al. "The Importance of Dietary Carbohydrate in Human Evolution." *The Quarterly Review of Biology.* 2015; 90(3): 251–268.

Morris, M. C., C. C. Tangney, Y. Wang, et al. "MIND Diet Slows Cognitive Decline with Aging." *Alzheimer's & Dementia.* 2015; 11: 1015–1022.

Ozawa, M., M. Shipley, M. Kivimaki, et al. "Dietary Pattern, Inflammation and Cognitive Decline: The Whitehall II Prospective Cohort Study." *Clinical Nutrition.* 2016; Jan 29. Pii:S0261-5614(16): 00035–2.

Ptomey, L. T., F. L. Steger, M. M. Schubert, et al. "Breakfast Intake and Composition Is Associated with Superior Academic Achievement in Elementary School Children." *Journal of the American College of Nutrition.* 2015; Dec 23: 1–8. Epub ahead of print.

Nuts

Bao, Y., J. Han, F. B. Hu, et al. "Association of Nut Consumption with Total and Cause-Specific Mortality." *New England Journal of Medicine.* 2013; 369: 2001–2011.

Bes-Rastrollo, M., J. Sabate, E. Gomez-Gracia, et al. "Nut Consumption and Weight Gain in a Mediterranean Cohort: The SUN Study." *Obesity (Silver Spring).* 2007; 15: 107–116.

Bes-Rastrollo, M., N. M. Wedick, M. A. Martinez-Gonzalez, et al. "Prospective Study of Nut Consumption, Long-Term Weight Change, and Obesity Risk in Women." *The American Journal of Clinical Nutrition.* 2009; 89: 1913–1919.

Carey, A. N., S. M. Poulose, B. Shukitt-Hale. "The Beneficial Effects of Tree Nuts on the Aging Brain." *Nutrition and Aging.* 2012; 1: 55–67.

Martinez-Lapiscine, E. H., P. Clavero, E. Toledo, et al. "Mediterranean Diet Improves Cognition: The PREDIMED-HAVARRA Randomised Trial." *Journal of Neurology, Neurosurgery & Psychiatry.* 2013; 84: 1318–1325.

Mozaffarian, D., T. Hao, E. B. Rimm, et al. "Changes in Diet and Lifestyle and Long-Term Weight Gain in Women and Men." *New England Journal of Medicine.* 2011; 364: 2392–2404.

Salas-Salvado, J., J. Fernandez-Ballart, E. Ros, et al. "Effect of a Mediterranean Diet Supplemented with Nuts on Metabolic Syndrome

Status: One-Year Results of the PREDIMED Randomized Trial." *Archives of Internal Medicine*. 2008; 168: 2449–2458.

Valls-Pedret, C., R. M. Lamuela-Raventos, A. Medina-Remon, et al. "Polyphenol-Rich Foods in the Mediterranean Diet Are Associated with Better Cognitive Function in Elderly Subjects at High Cardiovascular Risk." *Journal of Alzheimer's Disease*. 2012; 29(4): 773–82.

Valls-Pedret, C., A. Sala-Vila, M. Serra-Mir, et al. "Mediterranean diet and age-related cognitive decline." *JAMA Internal Medicine*. 2015; 175(7): 1094–1103.

Wengreen, H., R. G. Munger, A. Cutler, et al. "Prospective study of Dietary Approaches to Stop Hypertension—and Mediterranean-Style Dietary Patterns and Age-Related Cognitive Change: The Cache County Study on Memory, Health, and Aging." *The American Journal of Clinical Nutrition*. 2013; 98: 1263–71.

Beans

Darmadi-Blackberry, I., M. L. Wahlqvist, A. Kouris-Blazos, et al. "Legumes: The Most Important Dietary Predictor of Survival in Older People of Different Ethnicities." *Asia Pacific Journal of Clinical Nutrition*. 2004; 13(2): 217–20.

Shakersain, B., G. Santoni, S. C. Larsson, et al. "Prudent Diet May Attenuate the Adverse Effects of Western Diet on Cognitive Decline." *Alzheimer's & Dementia*. 2016; 12(2): 100–109.

Tsai, H. J. "Dietary Patterns and Cognitive Decline in Taiwanese Aged 65 Years and Older." *International Journal of Geriatric Psychiatry*. 2015; 30(5): 523–30.

Berries

Agarwal, P., T. M. Holland, Y. Wang, et al. "Association of Strawberries and Anthocyanidin Intake with Alzheimer's Dementia Risk." *Nutrients*. 2019; 11(12), Article 12. https://doi.org/10.3390/nu11123060.

Ahles, S., P. J. Joris, and J. Plat. "Effects of Berry Anthocyanins on Cognitive Performance, Vascular Function, and Cardiometabolic Risk Markers: A Systematic Review of Randomized Placebo-Controlled Intervention Studies in Humans." *International Journal of Molecular Sciences*. 2021; 22(12), 6482. https://doi.org/10.3390/ijms22126482.

Chen, X., Y. Huang, and H. G. Cheng. "Lower Intake of Vegetables and Legumes Associated with Cognitive Decline among Illiterate Elderly Chinese: A 3-Year Cohort Study." *J Nutr Health Aging.* 2012; 16: 549–552.

Devore, E. E., J. H. Kang, M. M. Breteler, et al. "Dietary Intake of Berries and Flavonoids in Relation to Cognitive Decline." *Annals of Neurology.* 2012; 72(1): 135–43.

Janabi A. H., A. A. Kamboh, M. Saeed, et al. "Flavonoid-Rich Foods (FRF): A Promising Nutraceutical Approach Against Lifespan-Shortening Diseases." *Iranian Journal of Basic Medical Sciences.* 2020; 23(2): 140–153. doi: 10.22038/IJBMS.2019.35125.8353

Kang, J. H., A. Ascherio, and F. Grodstein. "Fruit and Vegetable Consumption and Cognitive Decline in Aging Women." *Annals of Neurology.* 2005; 57: 713–720.

Khoo H. E., A. Azlan, S. T. Tang, S. M. Lim. "Anthocyanidins and Anthocyanins: Colored Pigments as Food, Pharmaceutical Ingredients, and the Potential Health Benefits." *Food & Nutrition Research.* 2017; 61(1): 1361779. doi: 10.1080/16546628.2017.1361779.

Miller, M. G., N. Thangthaeng, G. A. Rutledge, et al. "Dietary Strawberry Improves Cognition in a Randomised, Double-Blind, Placebo-Controlled Trial in Older Adults." *British Journal of Nutrition.* 2021; 126(2): 253–263. https://doi.org/10.1017/S0007114521000222.

Morris, M. C., D. A. Evans, C. C. Tangney, et al. "Associations of Vegetable and Fruit Consumption with Age-Related Cognitive Change." *Neurology.* 2006; 67: 1370–1376.

Nilsson, A., I. Salo, M. Plaza., et al. "Effects of a Mixed Berry Beverage on Cognitive Functions and Cardiometabolic Risk Markers; A Randomized Cross-Over Study in Healthy Older Adults." *PloS One.* 2017; 12(11): e0188173. https://doi.org/10.1371/journal.pone.0188173.

Nooyens, A. C., H. B. Bueno-de-Mesquita, M. P. van Boxtel, et al. "Fruit and Vegetable Intake and Cognitive Decline in Middle-Aged Men and Women: The Doetinchem Cohort Study." *British Journal of Nutrition.* 2011; 106: 752–761.

Poultry

"Eat More Chicken, Fish, and Beans." American Heart Association. Updated December 2, 2014 from heart.org/HEARTORG/HealthyLiving

/HealthyEating/Nutrition/Eat-More-Chicken-Fish-and-Beans_UCM
_320278_Article.jsp#.VxxI4KODGko.

Hurrel, R., and I. Egli. "Iron Bioavailability and Dietary Reference Values."
The American Journal of Clinical Nutrition. 2010; 91(5): 1461S–67S.

Fish

Larrieu, S., L. Letenneur, C. Helmer, et al. "Nutritional Factors and Risk of
Incident Dementia in the PAQUID Longitudinal Cohort." *The Journal of
Nutrition, Health, and Aging.* 2004; 8: 150–4.

Morris, M. C. "Nutritional Determinants of Cognitive Aging and
Dementia." *Proceedings of the Nutrition Society.* 2012; 71: 1–13.

Morris, M. C., J. Brockman, J. A. Schneider, et al. "Association of seafood
Consumption, Brain Mercury Level, and APOE e4 Status with Brain
Neuropathy in Older Adults." *JAMA.* 2016; 315(5): doi: 10.1001/jama
.2015.19451.

Morris, M. C., D. A. Evans, C. C. Tangney, et al. "Fish Consumption and
Cognitive Decline with Age in a Large Community Study." *Archives of
Neurology.* 2005; 62: 1849–53.

Schaefer, E. J., V. Bongard, A. S. Beiser, et al. "Plasma Phosphatidylcholine
Docosahexaenoic Acid Content and Risk of Dementia and Alzheimer
Disease: The Framingham Heart Study." *Archives of Neurology.* 2006; 63:
1545–50.

Olive Oil

Abuznait, A. H., H. Qosa, B. A. Busnena, et al. "Olive Oil Derived
Oleocanthal Enhances B-amyloid Clearance as a Potential Neuro-
protective Mechanism against Alzheimer's Disease: In Vitro and In
Vivo Studies." *Chem Neuro.* 2013; 4(6): 973–982.

De Alzaa, F., C. Guillaume, L. Ravetti. "Evaluation of Chemical and
Physical Changes in Different Commercial Oils During Heating." *Acta
Scientific Nutritional Health* 2018; 2(6): 2–11.

Estruch, R., E. Ros, J. Salas-Salvado, et al. "Primary Prevention of
cardiovascular Disease with a Mediterranean Diet." *New England Journal
of Medicine.* 2013; 368: 1279–1290.

Morris, M. C. "Nutritional Determinants of Cognitive Aging and
Dementia." *Proceedings of the Nutrition Society.* 2012; 71: 1–13.

Valls-Pedret, C., R. M. Lamuela-Raventos, A. Medina-Remon, et al. "Polyphenol-Rich Foods in the Mediterranean Diet Are Associated with Better Cognitive Function in Elderly Subjects at High Cardiovascular Risk." *Journal of Alzheimer's Disease.* 2012; 29(4): 773–82.

Valls-Pedret, C., A. Sala-Vila, M. Serra-Mir, et al. "Mediterranean Diet and Age-Related Cognitive Decline." *JAMA Intern Med.* 2015; 175(7): 1094–1103.

Wine

Estruch, R., E. Ros, J. Salas-Salvado, et al. "Primary Prevention of Cardiovascular Disease with a Mediterranean Diet." *New England Journal of Medicine.* 2013; 368: 1279–1290.

Lara, H. H., J. Alanis-Garza, F. E. Puente, et al. "Nutritional Approaches to Modulate Oxidative Stress That Induce Alzheimer's Disease. Nutritional Approaches to Prevent Alzheimer's Disease." *Gaceta Médica de México.* 2015; 151: 229–35.

Noguer, M. A., A. B. Cerezo, E. D. Navarro, et al. "Intake of Alcohol-Free Red Wine Modulates Antioxidant Enzyme Activities in a Human Intervention Study." *Pharmacological Research.* 2012; 65(6): 609–14.

World Health Organization. "No Level of Alcohol Consumption Is Safe for Our Health." Accessed March 31, 2024. https://who.int/europe/news/item/04-01-2023-no-level-of-alcohol-consumption-is-safe-for-our-health.

Panza, F., V. Frisardi, D. Seripa, et al. "Alcohol Consumption in Mild Cognitive Impairment and Dementia: Harmful or Neuroprotective?" *International Journal of Geriatric Psychiatry.* 2012; 27(12): 1218–38.

Valls-Pedret, C., R. M. Lamuela-Raventos, A. Medina-Remon, et al. "Polyphenol-Rich Foods in the Mediterranean Diet Are Associated with Better Cognitive Function in Elderly Subjects at High Cardiovascular Risk." *Journal of Alzheimer's Disease.* 2012; 29(4): 773–82.

Fatty Acids

Hill, M., R. Takechi, D. R. Chaliha, et al. "Dietary Saturated Fats and Apolipoprotein B48 Levels Are Similarly Associated with Cognitive Decline in Healthy Older Aged Australians." *Asia Pacific Journal of*

Clinical Nutrition. 2020; 29(3): 537–544. https://doi.org/10.6133/apjcn
.202009_29(3).0012.

Martinez-Lapiscine, E. H., P. Clavero, E. Toledo, et al. "Mediterranean Diet
Improves Cognition: The PREDIMED-HAVARRA Randomised Trial."
Journal of Neurology, Neurosurgery & Psychiatry. 2013; 84: 1318–1325.

Morris, M. C. "Nutritional Determinants of Cognitive Aging and
Dementia." *Proceedings of the Nutrition Society.* 2012; 71: 1–13.

Morris, M. C., D. A. Evans, C. C. Tangney, et al. "Fish Consumption and
Cognitive Decline with Age in a Large Community Study." *Archives of
Neurology.* 2005; 62: 1849–53.

Morris, M. C., C. C. Tangney. "Dietary Fat Composition and Dementia
Risk." *Neurobiology of Aging.* 2014; 35(S2): S59–S64.

Office of Dietary Supplements - Omega-3 Fatty Acids. Accessed April 1,
2024. https://ods.od.nih.gov/factsheets/Omega3FattyAcids-Health
Professional.

Ruan, Y., J. Tang, X. Guo, et al. "Dietary Fat Intake and Risk of Alzheimer's
Disease and Dementia: A Meta-Analysis of Cohort Studies." *Current
Alzheimer Research.* 2018; 15(9): 869–876. https://doi.org/10.2174/15672
05015666180427142350.

Teng M., Y. J. Zhao, A. L. Khoo, et al."Impact of Coconut Oil Consumption
on Cardiovascular Health: A Systematic Review and Meta-Analysis."
Nutrition Reviews. 2020; 78(3): 249–259. doi: 10.1093/nutrit/nuz074.

Zhu, R.-Z., M.-Q. Chen, Z.-W. Zhang, et al. "Dietary Fatty Acids and Risk
for Alzheimer's Disease, Dementia, and Mild Cognitive Impairment:
A Prospective Cohort Meta-Analysis." *Nutrition (Burbank, Los Angeles
County, Calif.).* 2021; 90: 111355. https://doi.org/10.1016/j.nut.2021
.111355.

Zhuang, P., Y. Zhang, W. He, et al. "Dietary Fats in Relation to Total and
Cause-Specific Mortality in a Prospective Cohort of 521 120 Individuals
With 16 Years of Follow-Up." *Circulation Research.* 2019; 124(5):
757–768. https://doi.org/10.1161/CIRCRESAHA.118.314038.

Vitamin E

Morris, M. C. "Nutritional Determinants of Cognitive Aging and
Dementia." *Proceedings of the Nutrition Society.* 2012; 71: 1–13.

De Leeuw, F. A., J. A. Schneider, S. Agrawal, et al. "Brain Tocopherol Levels Are Associated with Lower Activated Microglia Density in Elderly Human Cortex." *Alzheimers & Dementia*. 2020; 6(1): e12021.

Tanprasertsuk, J., T. M. Scott, M. A. Johnson, et al. "Brain A-Tocopherol Concentration Is Inversely Associated with Neurofibrillary Tangle Counts in Brain Regions Affected in Earlier Braak Stages: A Cross-Sectional Finding in the Oldest Old." *JAR Life*. 2021; 10: 8–16.

"Vitamin E." U.S. National Library of Medicine. Updated February 2, 2015 from nlm.nih.gov/medlineplus/ency/article/002406.htm.

B Vitamins

Johnson, L. E. "Vitamin B12." *Merk Manual*. Frommerckmanuals.com/home/disorders-of-nutrition/vitamins/vitamin-b-12.

Morris, M. C. "Nutritional Determinants of Cognitive Aging and Dementia." *Proceedings of the Nutrition Society*. 2012; 71: 1–13.

Wang, Y., C. Haskell-Ramsay, J. L. Gallegos, et al. "Effects of Chronic Consumption of Specific Fruit (Berries, Cherries and Citrus) on Cognitive Health: A Systematic Review and Meta-Analysis of Randomised Controlled Trials." *European Journal of Clinical Nutrition*. 2021; 77(1): 7–22. https://doi.org/10.1038/s41430-022-01138-x.

Wiedeman, A. M., S. I. Barr, T. J. Green, et al. "Dietary Choline Intake: Current State of Knowledge Across the Life Cycle." *Nutrients*. 2018; 10(10): 1513. https://doi.org/10.3390/nu10101513.

Flavonoids & Carotenoids

Charbit, J., J. S. Vidal, and O. Hanon, "The Role of Nutrition in the Prevention of Cognitive Decline." *Current Opinion in Clinical Nutrition and Metabolic Care*. 2024; 27(1): 9–16. https://doi.org/10.1097/MCO.0000000000001002.

Harnly, J. M., R. F. Doherty, G. R. Beecher, et al. "Flavonoid Content of U.S. Fruits, Vegetables, and Nuts." *Journal of Agricultural and Food Chemistry*. 2016; 54: 9966–77.

Morris, M. C., C. C. Tangney, Y. Wang, et al. "MIND Diet Slows Cognitive Decline with Aging." *Alzheimer's & Dementia*. 2015; 11: 1015–1022.

Neshatdoust, S., C. Saunders, S. M. Castle, et al. "High-Flavonoid Intake Induces Cognitive Improvements Linked to Changes in Serum Brain-

Derived Neurotrophic Factor: Two Randomised, Controlled Trials."
Nutrition and Healthy Aging. 2016; 4(1): 81–93. https://doi.org/10.3233
/NHA-1615.

"Vitamin A." *National Institutes of Health.* From ods.od.nih.gov/factsheets
/VitaminA-HealthProfessional.

Lifestyle Guidelines

"About Alzheimer's Disease: Risk Factors and Prevention." *National Institute
on Aging.* From nia.nih.gov/alzheimers/topics/risk-factors-prevention.

Barnard, N. D., A. I. Bush, A. Ceccarelli, et al. "Dietary and Lifestyle
Guidelines for the Prevention of Alzheimer's Disease." *Neurobiology of
Aging.* 2014; 35(S2): S74–S78.

"Color Additive Status List." FDA. Updated December 14, 2015 from fda.
gov/forindustry/coloradditives/coloradditiveinventories/ucm106626.
htm.

Dhana, K., P. Agarwal, B. D. James, et al. "Healthy Lifestyle and Cognition
in Older Adults with Common Neuropathologies of Dementia." *JAMA
Neurol.* Published online February 5, 2024: e235491. doi: 10.1001/jama
neurol.2023.5491.

Kawahara, M., M. Kato-Negishi, and K. I. Tanaka. "Dietary Trace Elements
and the Pathogenesis of Neurodegenerative Diseases." *Nutrients.* 2023;
15(9): 2067. doi: 10.3390/nu15092067.

American Association of Retired Persons. "Nutrition and Diet's Role in
Better Brain Health." AARP. doi: 10.26419/pia.00019.001.

Tip Sheets & FAQ

Asif, M. "Health Effects of Omega-3,6,9 Fatty Acids: Perilla Frutescens Is
a Good Example of Plant Oils." *Oriental Pharmacy and Experimental
Medicine.* 2011; 11(1): 51–59. doi: 10.1007/s13596-011-0002-x.

Baker, L. D., J. E. Manson, S. R. Rapp, et al. "Effects of Cocoa Extract and
A Multivitamin on Cognitive Function: A Randomized Clinical Trial."
Alzheimer's & Dementia. 2023; 19(4): 1308–1319. doi: 10.1002/alz.12767.

Dmitrieva, N. I., A. Gagarin, D. Liu, et al. "Middle-Age High Normal
Serum Sodium as a Risk Factor for Accelerated Biological Aging,
Chronic Diseases, and Premature Mortality." *EBioMedicine.* 2023; 87:
104404. doi: 10.1016/j.ebiom.2022.104404.

Dreher, M. L., F. W. Cheng, and N. A. Ford. A Comprehensive Review of Hass Avocado Clinical Trials, "Observational Studies, and Biological Mechanisms." *Nutrients.* 2021; 13(12): 4376. doi: 10.3390/nu13124376.

Elsayed, M. M., A. Rabiee, G. E. El Refaye, et al. "Aerobic Exercise with Mediterranean-DASH Intervention for Neurodegenerative Delay Diet Promotes Brain Cells' Longevity despite Sex Hormone Deficiency in Postmenopausal Women: A Randomized Controlled Trial." *Oxidative Medicine and Cellular Longevity.* 2022: 4146742. doi: 10.1155/2022/4146742.

Hecht, E. M., A. Rabil, E. Martinez Steele, et al. "Cross-Sectional Examination of Ultra-Processed Food Consumption and Adverse Mental Health Symptoms. *Public Health Nutrition.* 2022; 25(11): 3225–3234. doi: 10.1017/S1368980022001586.

Henney A. E., C. S. Gillespie, U. Alam, et al. "High Intake of Ultra-Processed Food is Associated with Dementia in Adults: A Systematic Review and Meta-Analysis of Observational Studies." *Journal of Neurology.* 2024; 271(1): 198–210. doi: 10.1007/s00415-023-12033-1.

Hersant H., S. He, P. Maliha, et al. "Over the Counter Supplements for Memory: A Review of Available Evidence." *CNS Drugs.* 2023; 37(9): 797–817. doi: 10.1007/s40263-023-01031-6.

Institute of Medicine. 2005. "Dietary Reference Intakes for Water, Potassium, Sodium, Chloride, and Sulfate" at NAP.Edu. doi: 10.17226/10925.

Martín, M. A., L. Goya, de S. Pascual-Teresa. "Effect of Cocoa and Cocoa Products on Cognitive Performance in Young Adults." *Nutrients.* 2020; 12(12): 3691. doi: 10.3390/nu12123691.

Porro, C., A. Cianciulli, and M. A. Panaro. "A Cup of Coffee for a Brain Long Life." *Neural Regen Res.* 2023; 19(1): 158–159. doi: 10.4103/1673-5374.375324.

Sachs B. C., B. J. Williams, S. A. Gaussoin, et al. "Impact of Multivitamin-Mineral and Cocoa Extract on Incidence of Mild Cognitive Impairment and Dementia: Results from the COcoa Supplement and Multivitamin Outcomes Study for the Mind (COSMOS-Mind)." *Alzheimer's & Dementia.* 2023; 19(11): 4863–4871. doi: 10.1002/alz.13078.

Sperling R., E. Mormino, K. Johnson. "The Evolution of Preclinical Alzheimer's Disease: Implications for Prevention Trials." *Neuron.* 2014; 84(3): 608–622. doi: 10.1016/j.neuron.2014.10.038.

Tan, T. Y. C., X. Y. Lim, J. H. H. Yeo, et al. "The Health Effects of Chocolate and Cocoa: A Systematic Review." *Nutrients*. 2021; 13(9): 2909. doi: 10 .3390/nu13092909.

Vyas C. M., J. E. Manson, H. D. Sesso, et al. "Effect of Multivitamin- Mineral Supplementation Versus Placebo on Cognitive Function: results from the Clinic Subcohort of the COcoa Supplement and Multivitamin Outcomes Study (COSMOS) Randomized Clinical Trial and Meta- Analysis of 3 Cognitive Studies within COSMOS." *The American Journal of Clinical Nutrition*. 2024; 119(3): 692–701. doi: 10.1016/j.ajcnut .2023.12.011.

Yeung L. K., D. M. Alschuler, M. Wall, et al. "Multivitamin Supplemen- tation Improves Memory in Older Adults: A Randomized Clinical Trial." *The American Journal of Clinical Nutrition*. 2023; 118(1): 273–282. doi: 10.1016/j.ajcnut.2023.05.011.

INDEX

brussels sprouts, 61–62, 64
buckwheat, 70–71
bulgur, 71
butter, 111–112
butter lettuce, 55, 57
buttercup squash, 62, 64
butternut squash, 62

C

cabbage, 54
California Olive Oil Council
    (COOC), 103
canned goods, 265–266
canned vegetables, 53
cape gooseberry, 90
Cardiovascular Health Study
    (CHS), 97
cardoon, 62, 64
carotenoids, 125–126
carrots, 59
cashews, 80–81
cauliflower, 62
celeriac, 59
celery, 59
cerebellum, 9, 11
cerebrum, 9
chayote squash, 62, 65
cheese, 112–113
cherries, 93
cherry tomatoes, 59
chia seeds, 81
Chinese eggplant, 60
Chinese long beans, 62, 66
Chinese MIND diet, 47, 49, 274–275
classic foods, in MIND diet, 254–256
coconut oil, 111–112
cognition
    definition of, 13–15
    function types, 14
cognitive decline
    and Alzheimer's disease, 19–20
    definition of, 15–16
    MIND diet, 31–33
cognitive health, 5
    aging, 42–44
    diabetes, 37–38

heart health, 36–37
mental health, 39–40
metabolic syndrome, 38–39
parkinsonism, 40–42
vegetables, 50–53
cognitive impairment, 17
collards, 56
cooked beans, 84
cooking, 146
corn, 66, 71
cranberries, 91
cranberry beans, 85
Creutzfeldt-Jakob disease, 18
crookneck squash, 66–67
cruciferous vegetables, 51
cucumbers, 67

D

daikon radish, 63
dandelions, 54
DASH diet, 27–28
dehydrated signs, 269
delicata squash, 62–63, 64
dementia
    cause of, 18
    definition of, 16–18
    symptoms of, 16–17
desserts, 230–237
    almond citrus chocolate bites,
        232–233
    choco-peanut butter cups,
        230–231
    creamy no-cook PB&J mousse,
        233–234
    greek yogurt with port wine
        reduction and walnuts, 236–237
    salgussam, 234–236
diabetes, 37–38
    type 2, 32, 37, 44–45, 69
    type 3, 37
Diamond Crystal kosher salt, 154
dietary antioxidants, 11
Dietary Approaches to Stop
    Hypertension (DASH) diet, 6, 25
*Dietary Guidelines for Americans
    2020–2025*, 39, 96, 108, 112, 121

dietary inflammatory scores (DIS), 38
docosahexaenoic acid (DHA), 12
dried beans, 84
dry pantry, 150–151

E

eggplant, 67
einkorn, 71–72
elderberries, 93
endive, 55, 57
endogenous antioxidants, 11–12
English peas. *See* peas
episodic memory, 21–22
executive functioning, 14–15

F

fall berries, 90–91
    barbados cherries, 90
    black crowberries, 90
    cape gooseberry, 90
    cranberries, 91
    huckleberry, 91
fall greens, 55
fall vegetables, 61–64
    acorn squash, 61
    black salsify, 61
    broccoli, 61
    brussels sprouts, 61–62
    buttercup squash, 62
    butternut squash, 62
    cardoon, 62
    cauliflower, 62
    chayote squash, 62
    Chinese long beans, 62
    daikon radish, 63
    delicata squash, 62–63
    garlic, 63
    ginger, 63
    hearts of palm, 63
    Jerusalem artichoke, 63–64
    pumpkin, 64
    sweet potatoes, 64
    turnips, 64
farro (emmer), 72
fats, 12–13
fava beans, 85
fennel, 65

fiber-rich beans, 262
fiddlehead ferns, 65
fish, 96
    choosing fresh, 99
    choosing lower mercury, 260–261
    fried, 97
    mercury in, 97–98
    types of, 99–100
flavonoids, 89–90, 125–126
    food sources of, 89
flaxseed, 82
folate, 51–52, 122–124
folic acid, 123
fonio, 72
food safety, 146–149
    leafy greens, 149–150
freekeh, 72
freezer, 151
French beans, 67
French MIND diet, 47
fried fast food, 113–114
frontal lobe, 10
frozen goods, 265–266
frozen vegetables, 53

G

Gai lan, 54–55
garlic, 63, 67
ginger, 63
global cognition, 21–22
The Global Council on Brain Health
    (GCBH), 249–251
glucose, 11
good and bad fats, 116–118
grape tomatoes, 67
gray matter, 15
great northern beans, 85–86
green beans, 65, 67
green soybeans, 85

H

hazelnut, 79
HDL cholesterol, 12–13, 38, 112
health nuts, 79–80
heart health, 36–37
hearts of palm, 63, 67
hemp seeds, 82

ACKNOWLEDGMENTS

This book is dedicated to my parents. My father, Dr. In E. Moon, is still a creative force to be reckoned with. He has big ideas and dreams he's working to realize to this day, and continues to serve his patients a few days a week. He's 82 with a biological age of 72. Meanwhile, my mother, Youjae Kang Moon, a chemist by training, is 82 with a biological age of 64. She sees her friends every week, spends times outdoors gardening and hiking the local hills, and still cooks her special brand of California-influenced Korean food every day, mostly from scratch.

If my father has shown me how to burn bright, my mother taught me how to be steadfast: learning every day, completing what I started, and doing it at the highest level of quality I can muster. Together, they instilled in me the importance of healthy food, being active, and always learning.

My partner in all things, Frederick Edward Gooltz, tasted every single one of the recipes in this book—many of them twice, some of them three times, as I fine-tuned them. He also made regular runs to the grocery store to pick up missing ingredients I needed for recipe R&D. Most of all, he brought joy and levity to the times I was able to step away from the writing or the recipes.

For support from afar, thanks go to my three sisters and our one little brother, Ahrie, Gurie, Suerie, and Kahmyong, on whom I know

I can depend no matter how far we are scattered around this earth (we cover three continents among us).

My aerial arts practice kept me sane and provided much-needed balance and joyful movement to combat the hours of reading research. I'm grateful to my coaches and training mates, some of whom I've been hanging upside with for more than a decade.

As ever, I'm indebted to the researchers who created and continue to study the role of nutrition in brain health, chief among them are the original MIND diet researchers.

I'm grateful to the Ulysses Press team, especially my editor Casie Vogel, who championed this second edition and provided a generous runway for me to review and synthesize all the new findings.

Last but certainly not least, this second edition has been made stronger by the feedback from the health professionals, community health workers, and individual readers I've had the pleasure of connecting with over the years because the first edition made an impact in their work and lives. I cherish these connections and can only hope the second edition earns its place on their bookshelves.

ABOUT THE AUTHOR

Maggie Moon (she/her), MS, RD, is a highly acclaimed nutritionist specializing in brain health. She is a Columbia University–educated, culinary-school trained, accredited registered dietitian with clinical training from top-ranked New York Presbyterian Hospital of Columbia and Cornell Universities. She has consulted with government agencies, national nonprofits, and global brands.

Moon is lead author of the Neurologic Disorders chapter in *Krause and Mahan's Food and the Nutrition Care Process*, a renowned resource in university nutrition programs worldwide. Additionally, she authored the Brain Health chapter in *The Culinary Medicine Textbook*, a comprehensive guide for community health initiatives. Her book, The MIND Diet, offers everyone practical nutrition solutions to enhance cognitive resilience through food for optimal brain health.

As a globally sought-after nutrition expert, Moon has shared her expertise with millions through international conferences, TV interviews, and publications such as *Eating Well, Good Housekeeping, Men's Health, Prevention, RealSimple, Well+Good, Women's Health*, and Yahoo! She is based in Los Angeles, where she enjoys hiking with her husband, cooking with her octogenarian mom, and creating content for @minddietmeals.